Statistics for Nurses
An Introductory Text

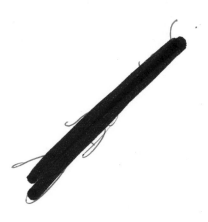

Statistics for Nurses
An Introductory Text

Frederick J. Kviz, Ph.D.
Assistant Professor
Epidemiology and Biometry Program
School of Public Health
University of Illinois at the Medical Center
Chicago

Kathleen Astin Knafl, Ph.D.
Associate Professor
College of Nursing
University of Illinois at the Medical Center
Chicago

Foreword by Harriet H. Werley, Ph.D.
Associate Dean for Research
School of Nursing
University of Missouri at Columbia

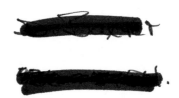

Little, Brown and Company, Boston

Foreword

Certain components of health care involve both art and science; this is true for nursing as well as for other professions concerned with delivering health care. It is, therefore, important that the science aspects of the professions be developed and implemented with increasing sophistication to generate research findings that are sound and defensible.

Nursing's heritage—stemming from Florence Nightingale, the scientist and humanitarian—dictates that nursing education curricula include method courses and opportunities for nurses to conduct and use research. The science of nursing will advance only through the gradual and continual accretion of new knowledge derived from valid research.

One of the most essential courses for the development of nurses as scientists is statistics. *Statistics for Nurses: An Introductory Text* provides students with the basics they need as consumers of research (that is, those able to comprehend professional and scientific literature). I hope this introduction to statistics will excite some nurses enough to seek advanced graduate preparation for careers emphasizing research and teaching. Such lessons are part of the process of sensitizing nurses to the value of research—one of the triad of teaching, service, and research on which all health professions are built.

This text gives a clear exposition of statistics and demonstrates its use as the basis for research and clinical judgment. Although it was developed for teaching statistics to nursing students, *Statistics for Nurses: An Introductory Text* is equally applicable for the wide range of students in the allied health professions.

Harriet H. Werley

Preface

Anyone who has browsed through the statistics section of a large university library might question the need for yet another introductory statistics text. At first glance it appears that a statistics book must surely exist for every possible need. Our particular need was for a text that would help our students to become knowledgeable, critical consumers of nursing research as well as prepare them for additional courses in statistics should they decide to pursue an advanced degree and a career in nursing research. But we soon discovered that such a book simply did not exist.

Because of the dearth of statistics texts for nurses and because of our own backgrounds in sociology, we selected a sociologically oriented text. For students that first quarter, the book only reinforced their conviction that statistics is at best tangential to nursing. The following quarter we changed to a "neutral" text, which, in place of sociological examples and problems, presented series of numbers generally devoid of any substantive meaning. Again the students were disgruntled. The second text confirmed students' suspicions that statistics is painfully uninteresting. In both instances, course evaluations from students cited the text as a definite weak point.

We subsequently undertook a systematic search for the "perfect" statistics text. The more evident it became that we were not going to find it, the more often one or the other of us would comment, "The only way we'll ever get what we want is to write our own book," until this became a serious intent rather than passing sarcasm. Eventually we did undertake to write the text that we had been unable to find.

While we do not claim to have achieved perfection, we hope that our book helps to bridge the gap that has existed for too long between the principles of statistics and the needs of nursing. It is largely based on lecture notes and class handouts developed for our introductory statistics course for undergraduate nursing students and is intended as an introductory statistics text for undergraduate students in nursing and the allied health professions.

This book is directed to the user of the "products" of nursing research—reports, journal articles, and the like—on the assumption that all nurses participate in research at least as consumers and that intelligent consumption is impossible without a grounding in statistics. It is not our intent to transform the reader into a "statistician." Our emphasis is on the interpretation and evaluation of statistical techniques and presentations. We deemphasize the more theoretical and mathematical aspects of statistics, which have minimal relevance for the practitioner.

Wherever we could, we have first presented techniques on a conceptual basis and then illustrated them by a presentation of short-cut computational methods with examples. The reader may be tempted to dismiss the conceptual presentations as hypothetical or irrelevant and jump ahead to the computational presentations. However, such a "cookbook" approach to statistics is strongly discouraged for two reasons. First, it will give the reader no appreciation of how to select the statistical method that is most appropriate for a given analytical problem. Second, while it is possible to become quite proficient at following a statistical "recipe," this ability is useless if not accompanied by an understanding of how to interpret the results of the techniques that are applied.

The book is divided into three major sections plus an introductory chapter and a concluding chapter. Part I, after a brief introduction to the nature of statistics and its role in nursing research, discusses methods of describing, summarizing, and comparing univariate distributions. Part II introduces the logic of statistical inference, the procedure for testing statistical hypotheses, and, finally, several of the inferential techniques most often employed in nursing research. Part III presents methods for examining relationships between two variables. The final chapter places the techniques discussed within the framework of the research process. In addition, an attempt is made throughout the book to integrate the material so that chapters build on one another and the reader is led to an overall appreciation of the nature and role of statistical inquiry in research. Our selection of statistical techniques to be included in this text was guided by our own reading of nursing literature, by suggestions from colleagues, and by Volicer's (1976) content analysis of statistical techniques reported in *Nursing Research* from 1971 through 1975.[1]

We spare the reader the arduous task of trying to muddle through long mathematical derivations (any interested student can find these in many statistics texts). However, we do assume that he or she is able to perform the arithmetic operations of addition, subtraction, multiplication, division, and simple algebra. The Review of Mathematical Operations in Appendix A is provided for those who need to review algebra.

Finally, since we believe it is impossible to understand statistics without practicing the techniques, we have included exercises titled Working With and Interpreting Data at the end of each chapter. The answers to the exercises are given in Appendix B. We strongly recommend that the reader do these exercises because they provide two kinds of experience. First, they provide practice in computational procedures; furthermore, because certain data sets are used repeatedly for various chapters, the student is able to observe how techniques build on one another and how different interpretations may arise

[1] Beverly J. Volicer. Statistical Index for *Nursing Research*, 1971–1975, Boston: Boston University School of Nursing, 1976.

from the application of different analytical techniques. Second, the exercises provide practice in evaluating and interpreting research findings selected from articles published in the professional journals. Part of being an intelligent consumer of research is understanding the process through which a researcher has arrived at his or her conclusions. Too often, the results of statistical analyses are treated as if they were mystical numbers whose origins are unfathomable to all but a select few. Knowing how to compute and interpret statistics oneself removes much of the mystery.

We gratefully acknowledge the contributions of all those who assisted in the creation of this book. We were initially encouraged to undertake this project by our colleagues, Jacqueline Haak Flaskerud and Janice Janken, and by Christopher R. Campbell, formerly an editor at Little, Brown and Company. Dorothy D. Camilleri, Alice J. Dan, Paul A. Reichelt, Maria Data-Sehr, Marikay Kieley, and Nena Sutker offered helpful comments on early drafts of the manuscript. Questions raised by students in our introductory statistics course at the University of Illinois College of Nursing were particularly valuable. We are indebted to many professional colleagues and predecessors, whose work is acknowledged throughout the text and in the bibliography. We commend Debra Bibbs for an excellent job of typing the manuscript. We also acknowledge the superb editorial assistance and support provided by Julie Stillman and Carmen Carrigan and their colleagues at Little, Brown. Finally, we wish to express our love and gratitude to Linda Kviz and to George and Ann Knafl for their innumerable direct and indirect contributions to this work.

F.J.K.
K.A.K.

Contents

Contents

Introduction

While Florence Nightingale is most often thought of as a great humanitarian, she was first a scientist and an astute statistician, as described in articles by Kopf (1916) and Grier and Grier (1978). More, even, than by a passionate caring and understanding for her fellow man, her work is characterized by the careful collection, analysis, and interpretation of the empirical evidence that she reported in her efforts to initiate social change. In fact, as a colleague of Adolphe Quetelet and Sir Francis Galton, two of the most prominent mathematicians and statisticians of her time and in the history of statistical study, she was a pioneer in the development and application of statistical methods to the study of social problems.

Since her time, the demand for and production of nursing research has grown enormously, especially within the last decade, as evidenced by the number of articles in the field published in an increasing number of nursing journals as well as in journals of related disciplines. A great deal of research is being conducted in clinical settings by administrators, clinical staff, and outside investigators, most notably university faculty and students. Although you, as a professional nurse, may not actually conduct a research investigation yourself, the chances are quite high that you will assist in carrying out and evaluating one or more such studies. Furthermore, nursing practice is increasingly becoming based on empirical research findings, and a working knowledge of basic statistics is essential if you are to evaluate knowledgeably the clinical applicability of these results.

It is important not only to understand what the results of a statistical analysis mean but also to assess whether the statistical methods applied are appropriate for a given situation. Therefore the main objective of this book is to develop your ability as an informed and critical consumer of research in nursing and related disciplines. Once this goal is accomplished you will be able to read most of the articles published in professional journals without having to skip over the sections describing the statistical methods employed and the findings of the analysis. But in addition to understanding most of what now probably appear as mysteries in those sections of research articles, you will be able to assess the appropriateness and quality of the analysis. A secondary objective of this text is to prepare those of you who may decide to pursue an advanced degree and a career in nursing research for additional courses in statistical methods.

What is Statistics?

The word *statistics* has two broad meanings. In one sense a statistic is a measured fact expressed as a number. The total number of residents of a city, the average number of children per family, the amount of change in a dietary patient's weight from one month to the next are examples of statistical information that may be generally referred to as statistics. In another sense statistics is a scientific discipline for examining, interpreting, and reporting research results, and it is this definition of statistics—as a field of study—to which this book is addressed.

Science in general consists of the formulation of theories to explain various phenomena, and the testing of those theories by empirical observation. The results of the testing may either support the theory or not. If they do not, the theory is then either modified or discarded in favor of an alternative theory, which in turn is also tested. A research problem is usually stated in the form of a question, such as "Are children of hypertensive parents more likely to be hypertensive than children of nonhypertensive parents?" The analysis and presentation of results in answer to such a research question is the major aspect of any research investigation. Statistics provides researchers with a logical, objective, and standardized system for drawing conclusions, in answer to specific research questions, from empirical data. Because statistics is based upon mathematical models, the possible biasing influence of the researcher's beliefs and expectations about the findings and their significance is eliminated. Furthermore the rules and procedures for each statistical technique are well defined, enabling others who might question a researcher's findings to reproduce the analysis and verify its accuracy.

Statistics consists of two main, closely related, approaches to the analysis of research data. *Descriptive statistics* covers methods for organizing and summarizing a set of observations conveniently and concisely by means of tables, graphs, and/or the determination of one or more representative characteristics or values, such as an average or a percentage. In addition to providing a profile of a single set of observations, an important use of descriptive techniques is to make comparisons. Such comparisons are made most often between two or more groups of subjects or conditions, such as a comparison between blood pressure readings for children of hypertensive and children of nonhypertensive parents, or a comparison of blood pressure readings of hypertensive patients under different dietary conditions. Another common type of comparison is between one or more sets of observations and a standard, such as a comparison between a patient's blood pressure level and a "normal" or "average" level for that type of patient.

Inferential statistics is a system of logic and computational methods for making generalizations or inferences from a *sample* of observations to a larger *population* of subjects or conditions which the sample is believed to represent. Because of such real and practical factors as time and expense, it is often not possible to study all persons or all conditions that are included in the scope of a research question. Therefore a researcher often selects a sample of the larger group of people or phenomena under study (called a *population*) from or about which data are collected. The researcher then analyzes these sample data using descriptive statistical methods to describe the characteristics of the sample. However, the researcher is not interested solely in the sample but rather in the entire population from which the sample was selected. He or she therefore attempts to generalize or draw inferences from the sample to the population. But, although most randomly selected samples will be representative of their populations, it can happen, although rarely, that a random sample contains an unusual and unrepresentative combination of members of the population. Thus, if the researcher is in fact dealing with such an unrepresentative sample, he or she will be misled when attempting to generalize from the sample to the population. Inferential statistics gives the researcher a means of specifying the chance or probability that he or she will be in error when generalizing from sample data to a population in a given situation.

Thus, when dealing with data from a sample, descriptive statistics is used to describe both the sample and the population, with inferential statistics providing an assessment of how confident the researcher may be in drawing such inferences from the sample to the population. For example, if the rate of heart disease is found to be higher among males than among females in a random sample of adults residing in the United States, the researcher would then like to extend this finding to the entire population of adult residents of the United States. But first, inferential statistics must be applied to assess the likelihood that such a generalization is an error. If the probability of committing an error is found to be sufficiently low, then the researcher will report that the rate of heart disease is higher among male than female adults in the United States with a specific (although small) probability that this conclusion is incorrect.

Scope and Approach of This Book

Although statistics is a mathematical discipline, this text does not demand an extensive command of advanced mathematical skills. We do, however, assume that you can competently perform elementary mathematical operations (addition, subtraction, multiplication, and division) and that you are familiar with *basic* algebraic procedures. Those who need to brush up in these areas should consult Appendix A, Review of Mathematical Operations, before attempting the following chapters. Most of the conceptual underpinnings of statistics, especially at the introductory level, can be understood in terms of common sense. Formal theoretical presentations are not necessary and are therefore not included in this text. It is not our intent to transform you into a statistician but rather to prepare you to participate in the exciting field of research as an intelligent consumer and, in some cases, a potential researcher or collaborator. Therefore, this book concentrates on the interpretation and evaluation of statistical techniques and presentations. There are many excellent texts that present this subject matter through a more mathematical approach. Some of them are cited at the ends of the chapters, and we encourage any of you who desire an exposure to a more mathematical orientation to statistics, or wish to pursue a particular topic in greater depth, to consult them.

As part of the effort to achieve precision and standardization, statistics has its own peculiar set of terminology that will make you think at times that you are taking a foreign language course. But most students become comfortable with these terms rather quickly. Statistics also uses certain written symbols and notation, along with formulas, which often appear threatening when first encountered. However, these are nothing more than tools that conveniently express concepts and procedures in a neat, shorthand manner. Indeed, much of the statistical mystique is dispelled once you become proficient in the statistical language. Although the verbal and written language of statistics is quite uniform, there is a slight variation in the statistical notation employed by different researchers and different statistics texts. The terminology and symbolic notation employed in this book are those that are easiest to understand and that are used most often by researchers.

The chapters are organized into three major sections whose topics are cumulative in the sense that they build on one another. Therefore it usually will not be fruitful to proceed with reading a new chapter until you are competent in dealing with the material presented in the preceding chapter(s). The first part gives descriptive methods for organizing, summarizing, and presenting a set of observations conveniently and concisely. Although this material is conceptually easier to understand than that presented in the other parts, Part I should be read with great care because there are fewer and less rigid rules for selecting an appropriate descriptive technique than an inferential technique. Therefore, although descriptive statistics may appear "simpler," it demands a more intimate working knowledge of its application and interpretation in various situations. The second part begins with an introduction to the logic of inferential statistics and then presents several of the most often employed inferential techniques.

5

Inferential statistics tends to be both conceptually and technically more demanding than descriptive statistics, because it involves an entirely new way of thinking for most people; careful rereading is suggested for those chapters. The third part presents several techniques for examining relationships between two variables, the focal point of many research investigations. This part combines descriptive and inferential statistics: a measure is first applied to describe the nature and strength of a relationship displayed in a sample and an inferential test is then applied to determine the generalizability of that finding to the population. Finally, the last chapter presents a brief integrative summary of the material presented in the previous chapters and attempts to place the role of statistics in research and clinical practice in its proper perspective.

Techniques are discussed first on a conceptual basis wherever practicable in order to show you how the data are manipulated in each case and thereby to help you understand when to apply them and how to interpret them. Where appropriate, this is followed by a presentation of shortcut computational methods with examples. The reader is strongly cautioned against skipping over the conceptual discussions, which may be incorrectly perceived as "useless theory," and jumping ahead to the computational presentations. Such a "cookbook" approach to statistics does not develop an appreciation of how to select and interpret the most appropriate statistical method for a given situation. The development of such an appreciation should be the goal of any statistics course, especially in these times when sophisticated electronic calculators and computers are often readily available to perform the computational tasks.

Although one may rarely perform a statistical computation as a consumer of research, a working knowledge of the process through which statistical results are derived is essential to intelligent consumption. Therefore students are strongly encouraged to complete the exercises included at the end of each chapter, in order to obtain experience in actually applying the statistical techniques presented. The answers to these exercises are presented in Appendix B.

Finally, we caution that a statistics text should not be read like the latest best-selling novel. Rather than curl up in a large soft chair in front of a fire with a glass of wine and wearing a set of stereo headphones, you will be well advised to read this book while sitting in a chair that provides firm support, in a cool, quiet, well-lighted room. This is because reading a statistics text is an active rather than a passive task. You should have a pencil and notepad handy to take notes, work through examples, and do exercises. It is especially important that you work through the examples as they are presented in the book

6

to verify that you fully understand how the results are obtained. Do not take it for granted that, because an example looks clear and simple, you understand it to the point that you could reproduce the example on your own. Above all, read slowly and carefully and do not hesitate to go back and reread sections that are unclear initially, several times if necessary. We hope that when you have completed this book you will agree with us that a basic understanding of statistical methods is not only intellectually challenging but very rewarding as well.

References

Kopf, Edwin.   Florence Nightingale as statistician. *Journal of the American Statistical Association* 15:388–404, 1916. Reprinted in *Research in Nursing and Health* 1:93-102, 1978.

Grier, Brown, and Margaret Grier.   Contributions of the passionate statistician. *Research in Nursing and Health* 1:103-109, 1978.

Descriptive Statistics

I

Variables and Their Measurement

Statistics are often impressive. In fact all that is required to win some people over to one side or the other of an issue is the presentation of a set of "statistics" that appear to favor the "desirable" side. But why is it that statistics so easily have an impact?

One apparent reason is that statistics is associated with *numbers* and mathematics, which generally are held to possess a great degree of accuracy, precision, and authority. However, there is nothing about any set of statistics that is sacred or makes it inherently correct. Statistics is simply a standardized set of analytical tools that are available to researchers who wish to examine a set of data. The finished product of the analysis process is only as good as the materials (data) used and the ability of the researcher to select the appropriate tool (statistical method) and apply it correctly. High-powered, sophisticated statistical procedures do not compensate for a faulty research design or careless measurement procedures.

This is especially important to bear in mind in our present computer-oriented society, in which researchers are sometimes mistakenly led to believe that data analysis consists of simply "dumping" the data into a computer. It is expected that the machine will, by some mystical process, provide an appropriate, complete, and accurate statistical analysis of the data, leaving the researcher the task of merely "writing up the results." The adequacy of such an approach to data analysis, however, can be quickly and easily evaluated by applying the GIGO Principle (garbage in, garbage out).

Just because we are presented with some statistical information, we should never believe that it is the absolute truth and final word on the subject. In order to appreciate why this is so, it is necessary to consider the process by which any particular set of statistics were generated. That is, we must understand where these numbers came from, how the measurements were made, and what they represent.

To that end, this chapter will review the most frequently used measurement methods and note some of the most common and serious sources of measurement error. An understanding of the methods by which measurements are made and the possible sources of error in them is essential to evaluating the reliability and significance of the results of any statistical analysis. Furthermore, different measurement methods provide different kinds of information, and the type of statistical analysis that may be applied to any set of data is highly dependent on the nature of the available information. We will accordingly distinguish between three levels of measurement and two basic types of variables. Finally, since

10
very few measurements are perfectly precise and accurate, we will discuss how measurements are often rounded before they are included in a statistical analysis, and the effect of rounding on the results.

Measurement Methods

The term *measurement* refers to any system of making and recording observations. The things that researchers try to measure are called *variables.* A variable may be generally defined as anything that may change in quality and/or quantity from one observation to another. It is precisely this changeable feature of variables that makes them interesting and important to researchers. All research involves an attempt to measure, describe, explain, and/or predict changes in one or more variables.

If a researcher intends to perform a statistical analysis of a set of data, the result of each empirical observation must be recorded in a numerical format. There are three basic methods by which this may be accomplished.

One method is by simply *counting* the total number of observations that occur in each of two or more categories. For example, each decade the United States Bureau of the Census counts the number of people living in the United States who are male and the number who are female.

A second, and perhaps the most familiar, method of measurement is the *application of a standard unit,* such as inches, kilograms, or degrees Fahrenheit. This type of measurement is usually performed with the aid of a standardized measuring instrument such as a ruler, a weight scale, or a thermometer.

A third measurement method is *ordinal ranking,* in which observations are arranged, either from low to high or vice versa, according to the amount or degree of a particular characteristic found in them. Observations may be ordered by using one of two approaches.

Ranks may be assigned according to an *objective* criterion such as the total number of observations that occur in each of two or more categories. The category with the most observations would be assigned the highest rank, and a lower rank would be assigned to each of the other categories according to the number of observations they contain, with the category containing the smallest number of observations receiving the lowest rank. For example, in an analysis of hospital patient reports on the kinds of information they want from nurses, if diet were mentioned, most often it would be assigned the highest rank. Similarly, if observations are measured by the application of a standard unit, the observation that contains the greatest number of units (pounds, for example) would receive the highest rank while the lowest rank would be assigned to the observation containing the fewest

11   measurement units. Thus, one might rank the birth weight of a group of infants from heaviest to lightest.

Another way of ordering observations is by employing a *subjective* criterion. In this case, instead of comparing amount or degree of a certain characteristic according to a frequency count or standard units, ranks are assigned according to judgments made by the researcher, by a group of "expert judges," or by the subjects being studied (assuming that they are human). For example, this procedure is used when people are asked to rank their order of preference for each of several alternative sources of health care provided on a list.

Many phenomena, especially in research involving human subjects, are not accessible to direct observation and measurement (e.g., patient satisfaction, marital happiness, and perception of stress or pain). In such situations the researcher must attempt to obtain an indirect measurement of variables by the use of *indicators*. Indicators are measures that are accessible to direct observation and that are considered by the researcher to be representative of the phenomena under study. For example, although patient satisfaction cannot be measured by direct observation, a researcher may examine certain measures that might be considered to be *indicators* of patient satisfaction. One possibility would be to ask patients to complete a "patient satisfaction questionnaire" during and/or shortly after a hospital stay. Another approach might be to record the nature and number of complaints about care made by each patient during a hospital stay.

Sources of Measurement Error

Except perhaps in the case of simple frequency counts, no measurement is perfectly precise and accurate. Therefore it is important to consider some of the major sources of measurement error.

First, it is essential that a researcher have a clear definition of any variable he or she attempts to measure. If the definition of a variable is vague, the researcher has no guide to determining the most appropriate method of measurement to use. If a variable has more than one possible definition, there may be an equal number of alternative approaches to measuring that variable. Also, the meaning of the research results may be interpreted differently by different observers depending upon which definition of the variable they employ.

Many concepts are highly abstract and do not have clear, concrete definitions. For example, there is no absolute definition of *health*. In such cases, the researcher must develop "working" or "operational" definitions to serve as guides for the measurement process. In the case of health, common working definitions usually deal with the nature and/or frequency of reports of how people "feel," the recognition and experience of symptoms, and the extent to which the performance of daily activities are unimpaired by physical or emotional problems.

Measurement error may also result from inadequacies or deficiencies in the measurement instrument. For example, a patient satisfaction questionnaire may not include the most relevant questions, or the questions may be asked in a confusing way; and a weight scale may not be calibrated or may be defective.

Since measurement is a human activity, all measurements are subject to error due to human fallibility. Observers may vary in many ways that may influence the accuracy or comparability of the observations they record. For example, observers may differ in their degree of alertness, temperament, intelligence, experience in using the measurement instrument, visual acuity, and so on. Also they often have opinions regarding the research topic and may have their own expectations of what the research results will or "should" be. There is a serious danger in such cases that the observers' opinions and expectations may influence the quality of their recorded observations. Researchers refer to this phenomenon as "observer bias."

Finally, many phenomena, especially human behavior, are very elusive and thereby difficult to measure. Attitudes and opinions may change rapidly and unexpectedly. Behaviors such as family and sexual relationships cannot be observed because it would involve an intrusion upon individual privacy. The observation of other phenomena, such as human development from infancy through old age, would be too time-consuming and extend beyond the life span of most researchers. And many phenomena, such as human attitudes and past experiences, are not accessible to direct observation.

Levels of Measurement

The measurement of variables is often referred to in terms of a series of *levels* that are distinguished by the nature and amount of information upon which the measurement is based. It is essential to understand thoroughly the difference between levels of measurement, because the selection of an appropriate statistical technique to analyze a particular set of data will depend to a large extent upon the level of measurement. We will be concerned with three basic levels of measurement: nominal, ordinal, and interval.

Nominal Level Measurement

Nominal level measurement distinguishes between individual observations in terms of differences in kind, or quality. This level of measurement does not consider the amount, or quantity, of a particular characteristic which is observed. Only the nature or type of the observed characteristic is considered. Observations that are identical or similar in kind are grouped together into one category for the analysis. Separate categories are established for observations that are different from those that were placed in the first category. Thus, each observation is placed in a category with all the other observations that are identical or similar to it regarding the characteristic being studied.

An example of a variable that is commonly measured on the nominal level is religion. A person's religion may be classified as Catholic, Protestant, or Jewish on the basis that each of these religions is different from the others in some sense. Thus, for the purpose of analysis, each individual will be grouped with all other persons who have the same religion. Similarly, the nominal level of measurement is employed when terminally ill patients' diagnoses are identified and each patient is placed into an analysis category with all other patients who have the same diagnosis.

The utility of the nominal level of measurement is limited by the fact that it provides the researcher with only a minimal amount of information about the observations being studied. All the researcher knows is that some observations are similar and some are different in a certain sense. The nominal level of measurement does not allow the researcher to determine whether one observation possesses more, less, or an equal amount of the characteristic being studied than another observation.

For example, knowing that a person is either Catholic, Protestant, or Jewish does not enable a researcher to determine whether that individual possesses more or less religion than persons who are classified in one of the other categories. Nor does the identification of a terminally ill patient's diagnosis provide a researcher with information that permits the researcher to categorize that patient as being more or less terminally ill as patients with different diagnoses.

Of course it often does not make sense to try to measure variables such as religion or diagnosis in terms of the amount of the characteristic possessed by an individual observation. Variables such as these might be considered to be inherently nominal in nature, since they can be measured only on the nominal level (or at least no one has yet figured out how to measure them in terms of quantity). For such *nominal variables*, the nominal level of measurement is extremely valuable, since it is the only way in which these variables can be measured.

Ordinal Level Measurement

When the way that a variable is measured not only distinguishes between observations that are different but additionally provides information on the amount of the characteristic being measured that is found in one observation as compared with another, we are operating at the ordinal level of measurement. Observations may be placed into categories with other observations that are not only similar in kind but also in which similar amounts of the characteristic being studied are found. The analysis categories can thus be ordered according to the relative amount of the characteristic found in the observations in each category. At the discretion of the researcher, categories may be ordered proceeding either from the lowest- to the highest-ranked category or in the reverse order, from the highest- to the lowest-ranked category.

For example, the ordinal level of measurement is employed when a researcher asks subjects to describe their health status as either very good, good, poor, or very poor. This method not only enables the researcher to distinguish between subjects in terms of whether their health status is the same or different, it also allows subjects to be compared on the basis of the relative level or rank of their health status. Thus, subjects who describe their health status as very good, feel that their health is better than those who describe their health status as good, poor, or very poor. Similarly, those who describe their health status as good feel that their health is better than those who describe their health as poor or very poor and so on. Other examples include evaluations of preoperative stress as low, medium, or high, and the classification of the condition of a patient as good, fair, poor, or critical.

Because it places observations into categories that may be arranged in order on a "more-or-less" basis according to the relative amount of the characteristic found in each observation, the ordinal level of measurement is very useful. It permits the application of what is called the *transitive law* in mathematics, which enables the researcher to make comparisons between observations indirectly by logically transferring information obtained through direct comparison of other observations. For example, to compare the height of two girls, Mary and Jane, we might stand them back to back and find that Mary is taller than Jane. We might similarly compare Jane with a third girl, Sally, and find that Jane is taller than Sally. We could then logically conclude that since Mary is taller than Jane, and Jane is taller than Sally, then Mary is taller than Sally. Thus, we are able to compare the heights of Mary and Sally indirectly by transferring the information we have from direct comparisons of both Mary and Sally with Jane.

The ordinal level of measurement is important because it is used frequently in nursing practice and nursing research. But although it provides the researcher with valuable information that is not available when the nominal level of measurement is used, the ordinal level also has certain limitations. While the researcher may know that a greater or lesser amount of a particular characteristic, as measured at the ordinal level, is found in one observation than another, the exact size or amount of that difference is not known and cannot be specified. This is because the ordinal level of measurement does not require measurements to be recorded in terms of standard units. As a result, although the researcher knows that different categories along an ordinal scale of measurement are separated by some interval, the size of the intervals between categories is unknown. Furthermore, the intervals between several categories located along a single ordinal scale of measurement are not necessarily equal in size.

Consider, for example, the classification of mastectomy patients into ordinal categories of "simple," "radical," and "extended radical," which are arranged in order from the least to the most extensive procedure. This classification system does not provide any specific information regarding how much more extensive (in a quantitative sense) a radical mastectomy is than a simple mastectomy or an extended radical mastectomy is than a radical mastectomy. All we know is that one is more extensive than the other to some unknown degree. We also do not know, nor can we reliably assume, that the difference between a radical mastectomy and a simple mastectomy is the same as that between a radical mastectomy and an extended radical mastectomy. Using the transitive law we can conclude that, since a radical mastectomy is more extensive than a simple mastectomy, and an extended radical mastectomy is more extensive than a radical mastectomy, an extended radical mastectomy is more extensive than a simple mastectomy. However, although the temptation is great, since we do not know the size of the intervals between categories, we have no basis upon which to conclude that an extended radical mastectomy is *twice* as extensive as a simple mastectomy. (It would similarly be invalid to conclude that Mary is twice as tall as Sally.) For all we know, that may in fact be the case. But it is also very possible that, if it were measurable, the difference is either something much less or much more than twice.

Interval Level Measurement

When a standard unit of measure is employed, and the size of the intervals between categories are known and equal, we are at the interval level of measurement. In contrast with the ordinal level, not only do we know that greater amounts of a particular characteristic are found in some observations than others, but we can specify how large the difference is.

Returning to the comparison of the heights of Mary, Jane, and Sally, instead of placing the girls back to back to observe height differences we might alternatively have measured each girl's height in terms of standard units of feet and inches. Suppose we did this and found that Mary is 5 feet 10 inches tall, Jane is 5 feet 8 inches tall, and Sally is 5 feet 2 inches tall. Instead of simply stating that Mary is taller than Jane, who is taller than Sally, we could have specified that Mary is 2 inches taller than Jane, who is 6 inches taller than Sally. Also, instead of concluding that Mary is taller than Sally, we could have concluded more specifically that Mary is 8 inches taller than Sally by means of the addition and subtraction of the standard measurement units.

Furthermore, note that if we place Mary, Jane, and Sally into height categories on an ordinal scale ranging from tall to medium to short and assume that the intervals between these categories are of equal size, we will be incorrect. This is because Mary, who is tall, is only slightly taller (2 inches) than Jane, who is medium. But Jane is much taller (6 inches) than Sally, who is short. Thus the size of the differences between categories is not uniform. Using the interval level of measurement, however, we find that the distance between the standard units, inches in this case, is constant. That is, there are no long, short, and medium-sized inches. Every inch is exactly the same size as every other, thus providing us with a standard unit of measure.

Other common examples of interval level measurements are temperature, which may be measured in degrees Fahrenheit or centigrade; weight, which may be measured in pounds or kilograms; and age, which may be measured in years, months, weeks, or days.

While categories are identified by the use of names to indicate a difference between observations in the case of the nominal level and by labels that indicate their relative position along a scale in the case of the ordinal level, categories on the interval level are identified by the value or amount of the characteristic found in the observations within them. However, just because numbers are used to identify categories of any particular variable, this does not guarantee that the variable was measured on the interval level. For example, burns are classified as either first, second, or third degree. But since it is not possible to specify quantitatively how much more severe a third degree burn is than a second degree burn, and so on, burn degrees are measured on the ordinal level, *not* the interval level. We could just as effectively distinguish between the severity of burns by describing them as type A, type B, and type C. A similar situation is patients' scores on a preoperative stress evaluation scale or students' grade point averages. Although numbers are used to indicate the relative position of observations along a measurement scale, if the numbers do not represent standard units of measure, we do

Table 2.1. Comparison of Characteristics of Different Levels of Measurement

Measurement characteristic	Level of measurement		
	Nominal	Ordinal	Interval
Differences in kind	Yes	Yes	Yes
Differences in rank	No	Yes	Yes
Differences in amount	No	No	Yes

not have interval level measurement. Therefore, we must be cautious of variables that at first appear to be measured at the interval level simply because numbers are assigned to identify categories, which are actually ordinal level measures.

As shown in Table 2.1, interval level measurement provides the greatest amount of information. All three levels allow us to distinguish between observations that are different from one another. Both the ordinal and interval levels allow us to compare observations by arranging them in order according to the relative amount of the characteristic found in each observation. But only the interval level of measurement provides the specific size of the differences between observations. For this reason the interval level is considered to be the most powerful of the three levels of measurement we have considered. Researchers strive to achieve a level of measurement that provides the greatest amount of information possible. If it is not possible to measure a variable on the interval level, then the researcher will attempt to develop an ordinal level measurement, usually considering the nominal level as a last resort, since it provides the least amount of information.

Most statistical procedures involve some mathematical operations, the most basic of which are addition and subtraction. Interval level measurement involves the rational assignment of numerical values to observations in terms of standard units of measure, which makes the use of mathematical operations possible. Therefore, as we will discover, the more advanced, sophisticated, and powerful statistical techniques require that the variable being analyzed be measured at the interval level.

The interval level of measurement allows the researcher to measure both positive and negative values, which are located respectively above and below a zero point. However, the location of the zero point on an interval level measurement scale is determined arbitrarily out of convenience and/or convention. It does not represent a true or absolute zero point in the sense that a value of zero indicates a complete absence of the characteristic being measured. For example, a reading of zero on a Fahrenheit or centigrade thermometer merely identifies a particular location along the measurement scale which is interpreted in relation to other values that lie above and below it. It does not indicate a complete absence of heat or temperature.

The lack of a true zero point means that comparisons between values measured on an interval scale are limited to descriptions of their relative positions and cannot be expressed in terms of a ratio between one value and another. Thus, it does not make sense to state that if the temperature outdoors was 30° F yesterday and is 60° F today, then it is *twice* as warm today as it was yesterday. Since there are many other possible temperatures that are even less warm than 0° F, all that can be said is that today's temperature is twice as high *above zero* as yesterday's temperature was.

However, when the measurement scale does include a true zero point, as when the weight of two children is measured in pounds, ratio comparisons are possible. Thus if one child weighs 30 pounds and a second child weighs 60 pounds, it is correct to state that the second child is twice as heavy as the first child. This is because the comparison is made with reference to a true zero point that represents a complete absence of weight.

When a measurement possesses all the characteristics of an interval scale but also includes a true zero point, we are at a fourth level of measurement, called the *ratio* level. Although the distinction between interval and ratio level measurement is important for many advanced statistical techniques, it will not be important in this book for three reasons. First, most measurements that possess the basic characteristics of interval level measurement also include a true zero point. Thus there are relatively few interval level measurements that do not also qualify as ratio level measurements. Second, interval level measurement satisfies the requirements of most statistical techniques frequently employed by researchers in nursing and related fields. Finally, and most importantly, interval level measurement satisfies the requirements of all the statistical techniques that we will discuss, and none of these techniques requires ratio level measurement.

Types of Variables

As you may have already realized from the discussion of levels of measurement, there are two basic types of variables: qualitative variables and quantitative variables.

Qualitative variables differ from one observation to another in terms of quality or kind. These variables are measured on the nominal level by some method of assigning observations into groups or categories that contain other observations of the same or similar kind. Patient diagnosis, race, and nursing specialty area are examples of qualitative variables.

Quantitative variables differ from one observation to

another in terms of quantity or amount. They are measured on the ordinal or interval level of measurement by assigning each observation a location on a measurement scale according to the amount of the characteristic being measured.

Variables that are measured on interval scales can be further distinguished according to whether they are discrete or continuous variables. Theoretically any interval measurement scale may be marked off in units of any size, from whole numbers, hundreds, thousands, and so on, to infinitely small fractions or decimals. Thus it should be possible for an observation to assume any value along the measurement scale—the only limitations being the precision of the measurement instrument and the degree of precision desired by the individual making the measurement.

Some variables, however, cannot assume all possible values along an interval measurement scale. Instead, these so-called discrete variables may be measured only in terms of specific measurement units. Family size is an example of a discrete variable, because it may be measured only in terms of whole units. That is, the size of any particular family may be one, two, three, or four members, and so on. Fractional measures of family size are not possible: we will never observe a family that contains one and two-thirds or two and one-half members.

Variables that may assume any value along an interval measurement scale are called *continuous variables.* This is because the scale used to measure them is marked off in intervals that may be subdivided infinitely; thus the continuity of the measurement scale is preserved rather than being broken into discrete units. Two common examples of continuous variables are age and weight. Although these measures are usually recorded in terms of certain standardly accepted units such as whole years and pounds, it is also possible to record them in terms of smaller, more precise units, if desired. In fact, theoretically, the intervals along the measurement scale for each of these variables may be subdivided infinitely.

The measurement of continuous variables is almost never an exact measure of the true value of an observation for two reasons. First, as we have already discussed, the accuracy of human measurements is threatened by several sources of error. Second, the task of subdividing continuous interval level measurement units to an infinite degree is impossible. Therefore, for the sake of practicality, the measured value of a continuous variable usually represents an estimated value which was derived by the process of *rounding.*

Rounded Measurements

There are three reasons why measured values may be rounded. First, as was just mentioned, values may be rounded because complete accuracy is simply impossible. Second, values are often rounded because the researcher's purpose does not require precision beyond a certain point. For example, if a relatively sensitive and precise measurement of birth weight is needed, the value may be recorded in terms of hundredths of a pound, such as 8.12 and 8.41 pounds. If less precision is necessary—for example, to make rather simple comparisons between infants—the value may be recorded in tenths of a pound, such as 8.1 and 8.4 pounds. Furthermore, if all that is desired is a quick or rough idea of an infant's birth weight, it may be sufficient to express the value simply in terms of whole pounds, such as 8 pounds. Third, values are often rounded in order to make mathematical computations quicker and easier. From the examples above, most people, if given a choice, would rather deal with values like 8.1 and 8.4 instead of 8.12 and 8.41 when performing calculations.

Measured values may be rounded according to one of three methods: to the nearest unit, to the last unit, or to the next unit. Rounding to the nearest unit is the method used most often in statistics and is also the method most familiar from everyday experience. Regardless of the method chosen, three basic steps must be followed when rounding a value. First, the rounding method that will be used must be specified. Second, the *rounding unit* must be specified. That is, it must be decided whether the value is to be expressed in terms of whole units, hundreds, thousands, tenths, hundredths, or whatever. This decision is based upon the degree of reliability or accuracy we believe is present in the measured value and the degree of precision we wish to express in the rounded value. Third, the measured value must be rounded according to the rules for the selected rounding method.

Rounding to the Nearest Unit

One of three possible procedures is used to round to the nearest unit depending on whether the value of the digit *immediately* to the right of the rounding unit is less than 5, greater than 5, or exactly equal to 5. Table 2.2 illustrates the use of those procedures to round each of several values to various rounding units.

Let us first consider the case of rounding the value 102.519 to the nearest tenth. The digit immediately to the right of the rounding unit is 1, which is *less than 5*, meaning that the value 102.519 is nearer to 102.5 than it is to 102.6. Therefore 102.519 is rounded to 102.5. Similarly, when 102.519 is rounded to the nearest hundred, the value immediately to the right of the rounding unit is a 0. Since 0 is less than 5, 102.519 is nearer to 100 than it is to 200, and the value rounded to the nearest hundred is 100. A similar procedure is used when the value 3020.358 is rounded to the nearest whole number and is rewritten as 3020.

Table 2.2. Demonstration of Rounding to the Nearest Unit

Measured value	Value rounded to			
	Nearest hundred	Nearest whole number	Nearest tenth	Nearest hundredth
75.697	100	76	75.7	75.70
102.519	100	103	102.5	102.52
254.012	300	254	254.0	254.01
462.500	500	462	462.5	462.50
513.555	500	514	513.6	513.56
3020.358	3000	3020	3020.4	3020.36

In contrast, when the value 75.697 is rounded to the nearest tenth, the digit immediately to the right of the rounding unit is a 9, and is *greater than 5*. Therefore 75.697 is nearer to 75.7 than it is to 75.6. The same procedure is used when rounding 462.500 to the nearest hundred (500).

If the digit immediately to the right of the rounding unit is *exactly 5*, one of two procedures is used depending on the value of the digits that are to the right of that 5. First, when rounding 102.519 to the nearest whole number, we observe a 5 immediately to the right of the rounding unit. But since at least one of the digits to the right of this 5 is greater than zero, the measured value is nearer to 103 than it is to 102. Similarly, when 254.012 is rounded to the nearest hundred, we determine that it is nearer to 300 than it is to 200, and 513.555, when rounded to the nearest tenth, is nearer to 513.6 than it is to 513.5.

But when 462.500 is rounded to the nearest whole number, all the remaining digits to the right of the 5 are zeros, indicating that 462.500 is exactly midway between 462 and 463. In everyday experience the usual practice is to round 462.500 up to 463. This creates a problem for researchers, however, because if that practice is followed consistently for a large number of observations, the rounded values will overestimate the measured values. On the other hand, if the researcher were to round such values down consistently (for example, round 462.500 to 462), the rounded values would underestimate the measured values. This problem may be avoided by rounding these numbers alternately down and up. The net result of this alternation would be that the tendency to overestimate the measured value by rounding up would be canceled by the tendency to underestimate it by rounding down for an equal number of cases. The convention that statisticians have adopted to achieve this effect is that, when rounding to the nearest unit, a number exactly midway between two rounding units is rounded to the nearest *even* number (thus, contrary to popular practice, 462.500 is rounded to 462).

Assuming that in the long run, for a very large number of cases, the nearest even number will lie below the measured value one-half the time and above it one-half the time, the desired balance will be achieved. Furthermore, rounding to the nearest even number often helps to simplify subsequent calculations further, since even numbers are "nicer" to work with because they minimize the occurrence of fractional results in common operations such as dividing the number by 2.

Rounding to the Last Unit

Sometimes measured values are rounded to the last unit, a procedure that is also often referred to as *rounding down.* Most persons are familiar with using this method of rounding in the reporting of age data. That is, in most modern Western societies, it is conventional to report one's age rounded down to the last whole year. Thus the true age of a person who reports his or her age as 22 years is actually somewhere between 22 and 23 years of age. Regardless of whether the person's twenty-second birthday was 2 days ago, 4 months ago, or 11½ months ago, that person's age will be reported as 22 years until his or her twenty-third birthday arrives. Similarly, using values from Table 2.2, 75.697 rounded down to the last whole number is 75, and 462.500 rounded down to the last hundred is 400.

Rounding to the Next Unit

Although it is a relatively rare practice, measured values may also be *rounded up* to the next unit. This method is often used in the recording of patients' temperatures. Since each degree on most clinical thermometers is divided into even decimals, it is most convenient to record thermometer readings in terms of even decimals. This is usually done by rounding the reading up to the next even decimal, or tenth of a degree. Thus a thermometer reading that lies anywhere between 99.2 and 99.4 would be recorded as 99.4. Similarly, rounding 102.519 up to the next whole number would yield 103, and 254.012 rounded up to the next hundredth would be 254.02.

Significant and Nonsignificant Zeros

Rounded values can be further simplified by distinguishing between significant and nonsignificant zeros. Significant zeros are important because they are necessary to preserve the location of the decimal point of a number and thus the size of the measurement unit employed. The use of significant zeros is illustrated in Table 2.2 where the measured value 254.012 is rounded to the nearest hundred and expressed as 300. In this case, the first two zeros immediately to the right of the rounding place, which is occupied by the 3, are *significant*, because they preserve the location of the decimal point at two places to the right of the hundreds place and thus preserve the size of the rounding unit. If, when 254.012 is rounded to the nearest hundred, the values 5 and 4 are not replaced with significant zeros, the rounded value will be incorrectly expressed as 3, in terms of whole numbers rather than hundreds.

On the other hand, note what happens when 462.500 is rounded to the nearest tenth. Since this value is already expressed in terms of tenths, with no remaining decimal values, the rounded number is simply 462.5. The two zeros that appear to the right of the rounding place in this case are not significant, because they serve no useful function. That is, if they are left off, the size of the measured and the rounded values does not change. Since it is much more convenient to work with a number such as 462.5 than 462.500, it is common procedure simply to leave off all nonsignificant zeros.

But it is important to note that not all zeros that appear to the right of the decimal point are nonsignificant. For example, when 254.012 is rounded to the nearest tenth, it is expressed as 254.0 in Table 2.2. In this case the zero that appears in the tenths place is significant and must remain in order to indicate the size of the rounding unit. Similarly, when 462.500 is rounded to the nearest hundredth it is written as 462.50. The zero to the right of the 5 is significant because it indicates that precision has been maintained to the hundredths place.

Rounding Error

As we have seen, rounded values are likely to be preferred to measured values because rounded values often help to simplify mathematical calculations. Although in most cases rounded values provide acceptable estimates of the values that were actually measured, they usually differ to some extent. This difference between rounded values and the measured values they represent is called *rounding error*. Table 2.3 demonstrates how the direction and size of rounding errors may vary depending upon which of the three methods of rounding is used.

When all values in a set of observations are rounded down to the last unit, the rounded values will be lower than the measured values. Therefore the researcher must remain aware that results derived from an analysis of values rounded to the last unit will most likely underestimate the size of the results that would be observed if the measured values were used. On the other hand, values that are rounded up to the next unit will be higher than the measured values. In this case the researcher must remember that the results of an analysis will tend to overestimate the size of the results that would be observed if the measured values were used.

Rounding error is minimized and is near zero when values

Table 2.3. Demonstrations of Rounding Error According to Rounding Method

Measured value	Rounding to last unit		Rounding to next unit		Rounding to nearest unit	
	Rounded value	Rounding error	Rounded value	Rounding error	Rounded value	Rounding error
4.1	4.0	− .1	5.0	+ .9	4.0	− .1
4.2	4.0	− .2	5.0	+ .8	4.0	− .2
4.3	4.0	− .3	5.0	+ .7	4.0	− .3
4.4	4.0	− .4	5.0	+ .6	4.0	− .4
4.5	4.0	− .5	5.0	+ .5	4.0	− .5
4.6	4.0	− .6	5.0	+ .4	5.0	+ .4
4.7	4.0	− .7	5.0	+ .3	5.0	+ .3
4.8	4.0	− .8	5.0	+ .2	5.0	+ .2
4.9	4.0	− .9	5.0	+ .1	5.0	+ .1
	Total	− 4.5	Total	+ 4.5	Total	− .5

are rounded to the nearest unit. Depending on whether the value of the digit immediately to the right of the rounding unit is below or above 5, the measured value will be rounded down sometimes and rounded up other times. The rounding error introduced by rounding some values down, causing them to be lower than the measured values, is balanced by the fact that an almost equal number of values are rounded up, causing them to be higher than the measured values. Since in most cases the researcher will prefer that the rounded values represent the measured values as closely as possible, rounding to the nearest unit is the method researchers employ most often.

For some variables, such as age, the method of rounding to be used is designated by accepted convention. But for the vast majority of variables there is no such convention. Therefore in most cases the decision regarding which method of rounding to employ is left to the researcher. If for some reason the researcher would prefer that the rounded values present a conservative estimate of the measured values, the method of rounding to the last unit should be selected. This is because, as we have seen, that method will underestimate the size of the measured values. On the other hand, if the researcher would prefer that the rounded values overestimate the size of the measured values, then the method of rounding to the next unit should be selected.

Another common concern regarding rounding is the matter of the selection of the rounding unit. This decision usually involves a trade-off between simplicity and precision. That is, as the size of the rounding unit increases (for example, from tenths, to whole numbers, to hundreds, and so on), the rounded value becomes easier to work with when it is included in mathematical computations. However, as the size of the rounding unit increases, the amount of rounding error also increases, thus reducing the degree of precision of the rounded value.

Also, when the results of mathematical computations are reported, the researcher must take care not to introduce an impression of greater precision than is warranted by the degree of precision maintained in the rounded values that are included in the computations. For example, a researcher may wish to report the result obtained when the measured value 10.463 is divided by 4. However, it is quite likely that the researcher may decide to simplify this computation by rounding the measured value to the nearest tenth. Thus 10.463 is rounded to 10.5. Dividing this rounded value by 4 yields the result 2.625. Since the original, measured value of 10.463 was expressed in thousandths (that is, to three places to the right of the decimal point), it may at first seem reasonable to express the result of this computation in thousandths as well. But it must be remembered that the value actually included in the computation was rounded and thus is precise only to the nearest tenth. To present the result as 2.625 would create an impression of greater precision than was actually available in the computation. This is because some precision was sacrificed when the decision was made to round the measured value to the nearest tenth. Therefore it would be most appropriate to round the computational result to the nearest tenth as well. Accordingly the result of 2.625 would be expressed as 2.6.

If greater precision is desired, the researcher may decide not to round the measured value at all. Dividing 10.463 by 4 yields 2.61575 as a result. But as before, this result suggests greater precision than was available in the computation to derive it. Therefore it should be rounded to the nearest thousandth and reported as 2.616. Furthermore it is important to note that this result *differs* from the artificially precise result of 2.625 that is obtained when the rounded value of 10.5 is used in the computation.

WORKING WITH AND INTERPRETING DATA

1. Identify the level of measurement for each of the following variables and justify your answer.

   a. Blood pressure
   b. Blood type
   c. Pulse rate
   d. Degree of pain
   e. Method of birth control

2. For each of the variables listed in question 1:

    a. Identify the variable as discrete or continuous.
    b. Identify the method by which measurement is obtained.
    c. Identify the sources of measurement error to which the measurement is subject.

3. On the basis of your clinical experience, identify at least one measurement used in nursing that is:

    a. *treated* as an interval level measurement but is *actually* an ordinal or nominal level measurement.
    b. *treated* as an ordinal level measurement but is *actually* a nominal level measurement.
    c. *treated* as a nominal level measurement but is *actually* an ordinal or interval level measurement.
    d. *treated* as an ordinal level measurement but is *actually* an interval level measurement.

4. Round each of the following numbers

    a. to the nearest whole number.
    b. to the last whole number.
    c. to the next whole number.

Number	*Nearest whole*	*Last whole*	*Next whole*
7.48			
12.52			
6.01			
27.805			
304.49			
9.50			

5. Round each of the following numbers to the *nearest* hundred and to the *nearest* tenth.

Number	*Nearest hundred*	*Nearest tenth*
5.53		
420.19		
1,359.98		

Grouping Data and Tabular Presentation

3

When it comes time to present their findings, researchers are typically confronted with an interesting dilemma. Having invested tremendous amounts of time and energy in a particular study, they are anxious to communicate their results to colleagues. And while these colleagues may be interested in the findings, they usually are not willing or able to sift through the mass of data a researcher has gathered during the course of an investigation. Thus investigators must temper their desires to report all the data with practical considerations of what will be most interesting and relevant to their potential audience. Even the most motivated, interested reader expects that the findings of a study will be substantially condensed and summarized before being reported.

This being the case, researchers need techniques for summarizing their data so that the reader is not unduly burdened by a mass of information whose overall meaning is not immediately apparent. In short, researchers need techniques that will allow them to simultaneously summarize and communicate their findings. This and the following chapter present a variety of strategies for accomplishing these joint tasks of summarization and communication. Their aim is to contribute to your ability both to understand and to critically evaluate research reports.

The techniques presented in this and the following chapter are applied to data from Knafl and Meara's (Knafl, 1974, 1976; Meara, 1976) study of La Leche League, a voluntary association that provides information and encouragement to women who choose to breast-feed their babies. The purpose of the investigation was to learn association members' ideas and practices regarding breast-feeding. In addition, the study asked for La Leche League members' views of the obstetrical and pediatric care they had received. Study data came from a variety of sources. During the pilot stage of the investigation, the investigators conducted intensive interviews with association members and attended association meetings. Using data from these sources, the investigators constructed a questionnaire that was mailed to a nationwide sample of association members. Of the 1,000 questionnaires mailed out, approximately 92 percent were returned. With the exception of Table 3.1, which is based on the total sample, most tables in this chapter are based on a subsample of 75 respondents to the questionnaire.

After a discussion of techniques for depicting qualitative or nominal level data, this chapter considers ways of summarizing and tabulating quantitative variables. That part of the chapter focuses on tables showing how measurements made

Table 3.1. Method of Birth Control: Entire Sample of La Leche League Members

Method	%
IUD	22
Condom	13
Foam, cream, or jelly	13
None	12
Diaphragm	11
Breast-feeding	9
Birth control pill	6
Sterilization	6
Rhythm	3
All other	5
Total	100%
Number of respondents on which table is based	857
Currently pregnant respondents	55
No answer	14
Total sample	926

on a single variable are distributed across a series of categories of that variable. For example, we consider data on a nominal variable, method of birth control, which is divided into qualitative categories such as IUD, birth control pill, and diaphragm. We then look at a quantitative variable, length of breast-feeding, which is divided into numerical categories such as 0–5 months and 6–11 months. Following this presentation of single variable tables, the chapter concludes with a discussion of cross-classification tables, which simultaneously classify observations on two variables. Regardless of the kind of table used, communication between reader and author is aided when the author clearly titles the table and labels its constituent parts. It is customary for table titles to include the variables depicted, number of observations on which the table is based, and the subjects or source of data.

Depicting Nominal Level Data

It is possible to present qualitative or nominal level data in tabular form. Table 3.1 shows the methods of birth control used by the women in the La Leche League sample at the time they responded to the questionnaire. In tables that show variables measured at the nominal level, the frequency with which cases fall into the various categories constitutes the *frequency distribution.* Like all tables, those depicting qualitative data are based on the number of subjects actually responding to a particular item. Thus, the percentages in Table 3.1 are based on the 857 respondents who answered the question "What is your current means of birth control?" The 14 subjects who did not answer this question are not included in the percentage base. Moreover, the 55 currently pregnant respondents were excluded from the percentage base. Although numerical frequencies are not included in the table, the reader can easily calculate these if desired because the percentage base (857) is included in the table. While there are no hard and fast rules for the ordering of qualitative categories, authors often arrange them in descending order from the category containing the most cases to the category containing the least. This procedure has been followed in Table 3.1.

In interpreting and evaluating frequency distributions of qualitative data, the reader should expect the researcher to state the *number of cases* on which his or her percentages are based and to *account for any discrepancies* between this number and total sample size. Classes should be *exhaustive*, meaning that each observation falls into a class, and *mutually exclusive*, with each observation falling into only one category. The reader might well question whether or not the categories in Table 3.1 are mutually exclusive, since respondents conceivably could have been using some combination of the birth control methods listed. This did, in fact, occur, and when it did subjects were placed into the category of the most effective method being used. Where categorization problems arise, the author should explain in the body of the research report the criteria used to categorize the observations, so that the reader is not left questioning the validity and meaning of the table. The reader should expect the author to communicate all the information the reader needs to interpret any tables presented in the research report.

Depicting Quantitative Variables

Researchers have a variety of techniques available to them for summarizing quantitative variables. In this section we will consider a number of ways of further condensing and tabulating the data presented in Table 3.2. In Table 3.2 the data—how long the subsample of 75 respondents breast-fed their infants*—have simply been recorded from each questionnaire with no attempt at further organization or summarization. It is therefore difficult for both the researcher and the reader to interpret the data. For example, it is not immediately apparent if the first respondent has breast-fed a comparatively longer or shorter time than the other respondents, or if nine

*Data presented are for first breast-feeding experiences of each respondent.

Table 3.2. Duration of First Completed Breast-Feeding Experience for Subsample of 75 La Leche League Members

9 mo.	2 mo.	15 mo.	6 wk	12 mo
3 days	3 mo	3 mo	9 mo	9 mo
2 mo	10 mo	3 wk	20 mo	7 mo
10 mo	12 mo	6 mo	3 mo	12 mo
6 wk	3 mo	13 mo	12 mo	6 mo
8 mo	9 mo	8 mo	12 mo	4 wk
6 wk	3 mo	3 wk	4 wk	10 mo
8 mo	15 mo	12 mo	9 mo	5 wk
6 mo	3 mo	11 mo	13 mo	14 mo
6 wk	12 mo	23 mo	21 mo	14 mo
12 mo	21 mo	2 wk	2 mo	12 mo
30 mo	3 mo	4 mo	8 mo	4 wk
5 mo	10 mo	8 mo	12 mo	8 mo
2 mo	10 mo	3 mo	21 mo	2 mo
42 mo	13 mo	6 wk	14 mo	6 mo

months is a fairly typical length of time for this group to breast-feed. Such comparisons are difficult if not impossible to make with the data in this form. Moreover, there may be certain patterns in the distribution that become evident only if the material is systematically organized. Further organization may indicate that cases cluster at certain points. Perhaps, for example, most respondents breast-feed less than six months. It is difficult to reach such a conclusion by scanning Table 3.2.

The Array

The data easily can be put in a more understandable form by constructing an *array*, a table that orders observations. Table 3.3 is an example of an array. In it the data have been ordered from shortest to longest breast-feeding experience. The researchers could also have ordered the data by beginning with the longest time span and moving to the shortest. In constructing an array, one has the option of beginning with either the smallest or the largest case. Although researchers rarely communicate data in this form, the array is the basis for constructing most of the tables and graphs discussed in this and the following chapter. Researchers usually construct an array as a first step in organizing their data for further statistical analysis.

Table 3.3 has definite organizational advantages over Table 3.2. The reader can easily differentiate extremely short from extremely long breast-feeding experiences. The two extremes, or range of the distribution of values, are now apparent (3 days to 42 months) and it is even possible to conclude that

Table 3.3. Array of Duration of First Completed Breast-Feeding Experience for Subsample of 75 La Leche League Members

3 days	2 mo	6 mo	10 mo	13 mo
2 wk	2 mo	6 mo	10 mo	13 mo
3 wk	2 mo	7 mo	10 mo	13 mo
3 wk	3 mo	8 mo	10 mo	14 mo
4 wk	3 mo	8 mo	11 mo	14 mo
4 wk	3 mo	8 mo	12 mo	14 mo
4 wk	3 mo	8 mo	12 mo	15 mo
5 wk	3 mo	8 mo	12 mo	15 mo
6 wk	3 mo	8 mo	12 mo	20 mo
6 wk	3 mo	9 mo	12 mo	21 mo
6 wk	3 mo	9 mo	12 mo	21 mo
6 wk	4 mo	9 mo	12 mo	21 mo
6 wk	5 mo	9 mo	12 mo	23 mo
2 mo	6 mo	9 mo	12 mo	30 mo
2 mo	6 mo	10 mo	12 mo	42 mo

someone who breast-feeds for nine months falls near the middle of this particular distribution.

Although the array represents an organizational improvement in the presentation of these data, it is still difficult to discern what, if any, patterns or trends exist among the 75 observations. Remember also that the original study included data from over 900 respondents. Most people would find an array with 900 entries unwieldy and overly time-consuming to interpret. Therefore, a method of systematically condensing these data into a convenient summary form is needed.

Ungrouped Frequency Distribution

Data organization and summarization are simultaneously accomplished when the investigator arranges the data in a frequency distribution. The frequency distribution is the most basic method of condensing and summarizing a set of data. Frequency distributions can be *ungrouped,* as in Table 3.4, or *grouped*, as in Table 3.5. In an *ungrouped frequency distribution* each of the observational categories is listed in a column. These categories may be ordered in terms of lowest to highest, as in Table 3.4, or highest to lowest. Once the categories have been listed, the number of observations or cases falling into each of these categories is recorded in a frequency column, labeled f. In contrast to an array, in which each category must be recorded every time it appears, the frequency distribution lists each category only once. While Table 3.3 contains 75 entries, Table 3.4 contains only 25. However, this is still a considerable amount of information to digest quickly and easily. Therefore the researcher usually

Table 3.4. Ungrouped Frequency Distribution of Duration of First Completed Breast-Feeding Experience for Subsample of 75 La Leche League Members

Duration	f
3 days	1
2 wk	1
3 wk	2
4 wk	3
5 wk	1
6 wk	5
2 mo	5
3 mo	8
4 mo	1
5 mo	1
6 mo	4
7 mo	1
8 mo	6
9 mo	5
10 mo	5
11 mo	1
12 mo	10
13 mo	3
14 mo	3
15 mo	2
20 mo	1
21 mo	3
23 mo	1
30 mo	1
42 mo	1
Total	75

Table 3.5. Grouped Frequency Distribution of First Breast-Feeding Experience for a Subsample of 75 La Leche League Members

Class interval	f
0– 5 mo	28
6–11 mo	22
12–17 mo	18
18–23 mo	5
24–29 mo	0
30–35 mo	1
36–41 mo	0
42–47 mo	1
Total	75

Table 3.6. Grouped Frequency Distribution of First Breast-Feeding Experience for Subsample of 75 La Leche League Members

Class interval	f
0- 5	28
6-11	22
12-17	18
> 17	7
Total	75

carries the summarization process a step further and con-
structs a grouped frequency distribution.

Grouped Frequency Distribution

Tables 3.5 and 3.6 are examples of grouped frequency distributions. They both present the same data as in the array and
ungrouped frequency distribution, but the data are now
grouped into a series of class intervals of which each contains
a number of the individual categories. Table 3.5 contains eight
class intervals (0-5, 6-11, 12-17, etc.). Table 3.6 contains
four class intervals with the last class of > 17 (greater than 17)
being an open class, since its upper boundary has not been
specified. Researchers sometimes use open classes as either the
first or last class interval of a frequency distribution. While
this practice may preclude certain further analytic steps, it is
useful when there are wide gaps in the distribution of cases.
Since the data have been condensed, a grouped frequency distribution facilitates the identification of trends and patterns
in the data. However, some of the detailed information about
the *exact* value of each observation, which remains available
in an array or an ungrouped frequency distribution, is lost
in the process of combining categories for a grouped distribution.

CONSTRUCTING A GROUPED FREQUENCY DISTRIBUTION
The researcher who wants to present data in the form of a
grouped frequency distribution first has to determine the
number and size of the classes into which the data will be
grouped. This involves balancing the aim of condensing data
with the desire to convey the data fully. With any set of data,
as the researcher reduces the number of class intervals in the
frequency distribution, she or he simultaneously reduces the
amount of information communicated.

For example, less information is lost in Table 3.5 than in
Table 3.6. As the class intervals increase in size or width, less
information is communicated as to the distribution of the
data across the range of categories. When presented with a

grouped frequency distribution, the reader has no way of knowing exactly how many, if any, cases fell into a given category. He or she only knows the number of cases falling into the range of categories encompassed by the class interval.

There are no hard and fast rules for the researcher to follow in determining the number of classes appropriate to his or her set of data. Although some texts list specific guidelines as to the minimum and maximum number of classes in a frequency distribution, these vary considerably from author to author. Clearly the crucial issue is not the number of categories per se but the adequacy of the information communicated. The researcher wants to avoid both distorting the data and burdening the reader with unnecessary detail.

In the end, it is up to you, the reader, to decide if a given frequency distribution effectively communicates the data. One way to do this is to compare your interpretation of a table with that of the author. Tables and graphs should communicate sufficient data so the reader can draw his or her own conclusions about the research results, before consulting the text. This is especially crucial in an applied science such as nursing, where the reader is often a clinician who wants to determine the meaning of the data for his or her particular setting. The data may have different implications and mean different things to different people. An optimally detailed table both facilitates communication and encourages further interpretation and application of the data.

Although the optimal number of categories needed to communicate the data to the reader will vary considerably depending on the nature of the study, some well-established conventions do exist for constructing a grouped frequency distribution. Investigators facilitate communication when the range of values covered in each class interval is uniform. Unless the investigator has some special reason or purpose for establishing classes of unequal size, it is generally considered poor form to do so, because this practice may confuse the interpretation of the data. The use of open classes is an exception to this general guideline. As noted in connection with Table 3.6, the use of open classes is appropriate when there are large gaps in the distribution of cases and further analysis of the data is not being undertaken. As with qualitative class categories, these intervals should be exhaustive, accommodating all the data, and mutually exclusive, categorizing each observation into only one category. For example, the class intervals in Tables 3.4 and 3.5 would not have been exhaustive if there had been an observation of 60 months, since this case would not have fit into any of the categories. On the other hand the following is an example of categories that are not mutually exclusive, since they overlap: 0-5, 5-10, 10-15, 15-20. When categories overlap, it is impossible to categorize certain observations. For example, does someone who breast-fed for 5 months belong in the first or second category? In constructing and evaluating tables, one should remember the rules of exhaustiveness and mutual exclusivity.

Class intervals are typically recorded as rounded numbers. This is the case in Table 3.5, in which observations were rounded to the nearest whole month. Recalling the rules of rounding discussed in the previous chapter, the *true* as opposed to the *rounded* limits for Table 3.5 would be as follows:

Rounded class limits	True class limits
0- 5	—.5- 5.5
6-11	5.5-11.5
12-17	11.5-17.5
18-23	17.5-23.5
24-29	23.5-29.5
30-35	29.5-35.5
36-41	35.5-41.5
42-47	41.5-47.5

Two things about the true limits of these categories may seem confusing. First, they seem to violate the rule that categories should be mutually exclusive, since the upper boundary or limit of one category is the lower limit or boundary of the next. What happens, then, when the investigator tries to classify the case of someone who has breast-fed 5.5 months? When the observations are rounded to the nearest whole month, this ceases to be an issue, because an observation of 5.5 is rounded to 6, the nearest *even* number. Similarly, 11.5 would be rounded to 12, and so on. Thus the 6–11 interval under rounded limits includes observations that lie between 5.5 and *up to but not including* 11.5. A second confusing aspect of the true limits of class intervals is that they sometimes violate the nature of reality. Common sense tells us that no one breast-feeds for —.5 months. When we are working with true class limits, however, statistical sense and convention take precedent over common sense and we maintain the negative lower limit of the first class interval. The importance of this distinction between the rounded limits and the true limits of a class will become apparent in Chapter 5. Finally, it is also usual, although not absolutely mandatory, for the author to list categories in ascending order, starting with the lowest and going to the highest values.

Once the author has established his or her class intervals, it is a simple process to tally the cases into the appropriate interval. Table 3.7 illustrates the simple process by which the data in Table 3.6 were summarized in a grouped frequency distribution. If the data have been organized into any array, the tallying process is greatly simplified.

Table 3.7. Constructing a Grouped Frequency Distribution of Duration of First Breast-Feeding Experience for a Subsample of 75 La Leche League Members

Class interval	Tally	f
0- 5	~~HHH~~ ~~HHH~~ ~~HHH~~ ~~HHH~~ ~~HHH~~ 111	28
6-11	~~HHH~~ ~~HHH~~ ~~HHH~~ ~~HHH~~ 11	22
12-17	~~HHH~~ ~~HHH~~ ~~HHH~~ 111	18
> 17	~~HHH~~ 11	7
	Total	75

The use of such phrases as "statistical convention" and "usual practice" illustrates another point about table construction. In general, the process is governed by a set of standard operating procedures, usual ways of doing things. Innovative efforts on the author's part are more likely to obscure than facilitate communication. Thus, although imagination and creativity are generally assets to the researcher, they often are best held in abeyance when presenting data in tabular form, since standard convention will be more readily understandable to the reader.

PERCENTAGED GROUPED FREQUENCY DISTRIBUTION
The researcher may choose to depict class frequencies in terms of percentages. Such a conversion facilitates the comparison of frequency distributions of unequal sizes. For example, we might have wanted to compare La Leche League members' breast-feeding experiences with the experiences of women who do not belong to the organization. If we had collected data from 100 nonmembers of the organization, it would have been difficult to compare this with the information from the over 900 organization members without first converting the raw numbers to percentages. For example, for one given category— like 12-17 months—each of these two hypothetical distributions of cases might contain the same number of 10 observations. This does not mean, however, that the two distributions are actually equivalent in that category. In the sample of 100 nonmembers, 10 observations constitutes 10 percent of the total number of cases. For the sample of 900 La Leche League members, 10 observations is approximately one percent of the cases. Thus in spite of identical numerical frequencies, *proportionately* fewer of the members as compared to the nonmembers would have fallen into this category.

It is a simple task for either the reader or the researcher to make such a conversion. For example, to determine the percentage of cases that fall into the 0-5 category in Table 3.6 we divide 28, the number of cases in that category, by 75, the

Table 3.8. Percentaged Grouped Frequency Distribution of Duration of First Breast-Feeding Experience for Subsample of 75 La Leche League Members

Class interval	f	%
0- 5 mo	28	37
6-11 mo	22	29
12-17 mo	18	24
> 17	7	9
Totals 75		99%

total number of cases in the table. This process yields the decimal figure or proportion of .37. By multiplying .37 by 100 we can convert the figure to a percentage. Table 3.8 is a percentaged grouped frequency distribution. The percentage column should total approximately 100. When it does not, as in Table 3.8, where the percentage column totals 99 percent, this is the cumulative result of rounding error in figuring percentages for individual class intervals.

It is especially appropriate for investigators to convert table frequencies to percentages when they are comparing sets of data from an unequal number of cases. Even if the researcher has failed to convert frequencies to percentages, it is a relatively simple task for the reader to perform. Moreover, you may want to make such a conversion on your own in order to compare data from several research projects or reports.

Cumulative Frequency Distributions

Grouped frequency distributions can easily be converted to cumulative distributions such as those depicted in Tables 3.9 and 3.10. By showing how many or what percentage of cases fall above (*more-than* cumulative distribution) or below (*less-than* cumulative distribution) a certain point, cumulative frequency tables communicate more information to the reader than a grouped frequency distribution does.

A more-than cumulative table indicates the number or percentage of cases falling *above* the *lower true class limit* for each class interval. Thus Table 3.9 shows the number of respondents who breast-fed longer than —.5, 5.5, 11.5, 17.5, 23.5, 29.5, 35.5, and 41.5 months, since these are the true lower class limits for each class interval. Reading this table, we can see, for example, that 25 subjects, or one-third of the sample, breast-fed for more than 11.5 months; seven subjects or approximately 10 percent of the sample breast-fed for over 17.5 months.

In contrast the less-than cumulative table communicates the number or percentage of respondents falling *below* the *upper*

Table 3.9. *More-Than* Cumulative Frequency Distribution of Duration of First Completed Breast-Feeding Experience for Subsample of 75 La Leche League Members

Duration	f	Cumulative f	Cumulative %
0- 5 mo	28	75	100
6-11 mo	22	47	63
12-17 mo	18	25	33
18-23 mo	5	7	9
24-29 mo	0	2	3
30-35 mo	1	2	3
36-41 mo	0	1	1
42-47 mo	1	1	1
	N=75		

Table 3.10. *Less-Than* Cumulative Frequency Distribution of Duration of First Completed Breast-Feeding Experience for Subsample of 75 La Leche League Members

Duration	f	Cumulative f	Cumulative %
0- 5 mo	28	28	37
6-11 mo	22	50	67
12-17 mo	18	68	91
18-23 mo	5	73	97
24-29 mo	0	73	97
30-35 mo	1	74	99
36-41 mo	0	74	99
42-47 mo	1	75	100

true class limit of each class interval. Thus Table 3.10 lists the number of women breast-feeding less than 47.5, 41.5, 35.5, 29.5, 23.5, 17.5, 11.5, and 5.5 months, these being the upper true limits of each class interval. By looking at Table 3.10 we can see that 68 subjects breast-fed less than 17.5 months; 50 subjects breast-fed for less than 11.5 months. In order to read and interpret such cumulative distributions correctly, the reader must remember that the *lower* true class limit is the point of reference for a more-than cumulative table, and the *upper* true class limit is the point of reference for the less-than table.

More-than and less-than cumulative tables represent opposite sides of the same coin as far as communicating data. Researchers select one or the other in depicting a particular set of data, depending on which method is best suited to the purpose at hand. The decision as to which form is more appropriate is based on what characteristic of the data the researcher wishes to emphasize. Moreover it is possible for researchers to construct cumulative percentage distributions. Like any percentage distribution, these facilitate comparison between two groups or samples of unequal size.

Cumulative frequency or percentage distributions can facilitate comparisons between sets of data. For example, it might be interesting to compare the percentages of La Leche League members and nonmembers who breast-fed for a year or more or who breast-fed for less than 6 months.

Constructing a Cumulative Distribution

It is a relatively simple matter to transform a simple frequency distribution into a cumulative one. To convert Table 3.5 into the more-than cumulative distribution shown in Table 3.9, one would simply successively cumulate or add cases, moving from the number of cases in the highest class interval (42–47) through the number of cases in the lowest class interval (0–5). Starting with the 42–47 month interval we see that we have one subject. The next step is to add to this case the number of subjects in the 36–41 range. Since no observations fell into this category, we have still a cumulated frequency of 1 at this point. Moving to the 30–35 class interval, we see that one subject fell into this class. Adding this to the one subject who fell above this point, we have accumulated two individuals who breast-fed more than 29.5 months, the lower true class limit of the category. No additional cases are added in the 24–29 class interval; the cumulative frequency remains 2. However 5 cases fell into the 18–23 interval, bringing our cumulated frequency to 7. Moving to the next category we add an additional 18 cases to the 7 already accumulated and record that 25 subjects breast-fed for more than 11.5 months. Adding the 22 cases in the 6–11 category to the 25 we have already cumulated, we see that 47 subjects have breast-fed for more than 5.5 months, the lower true limit of the 6–11 class interval. Adding the final 28 cases that fall into the first class interval we have cumulated all 75 cases.

The process for converting Table 3.5 to the less-than cumulative frequency distribution in Table 3.10 is the same as that just described for a more-than cumulation, except that cases are cumulated in the opposite direction, moving from the lowest through the highest class interval. Using the upper true limit of the class as a reference point, we have accumulated 28 subjects who have breast-fed for 5.5 months or less. To find out how many subjects have breast-fed for less than 11.5 months, we add the number of cases in the first and second class intervals and obtain a cumulated frequency of 50. If we wanted to know how many respondents had breast-fed for less than 23.5 months, we would cumulate the number or percentage of subjects in the first four class intervals.

Cross-Classification

The tabular presentations discussed so far have shown the distribution of one variable, which has been divided into a number of categories. Specifically, we have looked at tables that have presented data on one variable: either the duration of breast-feeding experience or the method of birth control. It is also possible for researchers to classify observations according to two or more dimensions simultaneously. The resulting table is called a *cross-classification*. Table 3.11, based on hypothetical data, is an example of a cross-classification table. Although Table 3.11 comprises one quantitative variable (number of months) and one qualitative variable (membership), cross-classifications can be constructed when both variables are either quantitative or qualitative.

By depicting the comparative frequency or *joint occurrence* of variables, cross-classifications can provide insights into how variables may be related. This particular purpose is better served when frequencies are converted to percentages. For example, in Table 3.12 the frequencies in Table 3.11 have

Table 3.11. Cross-Classification of Duration of Breast-Feeding Experience by La Leche League Membership

	Months				
Membership	*0–5*	*6–11*	*12–17*	*18–23*	*Total*
Yes	7	21	37	35	100
No	15	31	4	0	50
Total	22	52	41	35	150

Table 3.12. Percentage Cross-Classification of Duration of First Breast-Feeding Experience by La Leche League Membership

Membership	Months				*Total*
	0–5	*6–11*	*12–17*	*18–23*	*(%)*
Yes	5	14	25	23	67
No	10	21	3	0	33
Total (%)	15	35	27	23	100
Number of respondents = 150					

been converted to percentages based on the total number of observations in the table ($N = 150$).

Percentages based on a small number of cases can be unreliable because they are not very stable. For example, if we had a group of ten subjects and nine of them were La Leche League members, this would constitute a 90 percent membership rate. However, a shift of only one subject either into or out of the membership category would result in a change of 10 percentage points. The magnitude of the percentage change is a function of the small total number of cases. In contrast, in a sample of 100, a shift of one observation into or out of a category would result in a much smaller percentage difference of 1 percent. The researcher should, therefore, always report the base number from which the percentages were computed. As a reader, you might view the data in Table 3.12 quite differently if it were based on 25 observations instead of 150.

Researchers use a different strategy in constructing a cross-classification when they want to explore the possibility that one variable causally influences another. In this case each category of the independent or causal variable is totaled to 100 percent as in Table 3.13, in which membership is treated as the independent variable. Note that this table includes the actual number of cases for each category of the independent variable, so the reader is apprised of the bases of the table percentages. When the independent variable is listed along the left-hand side of the table (as in this example), each row will total 100 percent. When the independent variable has been listed across the top of the table, each column will total 100 percent.

In order to interpret a cross-classification such as this, the reader must know which variable the author is treating as the independent variable and which as the dependent variable. While that should be clearly specified in the body of the article, it is also possible to determine it from the table, since each category of the independent variable totals to 100 percent.

In constructing Table 3.13 as we have, we are asking, "Does membership in this organization influence how long a woman

Table 3.13. Cross-Classification of Duration of Breast-Feeding Experience by La Leche League Membership

Membership	Months				Total (%)	N
	0–5	6–11	12–17	18–23		
Yes	7	21	37	35	100	100
No	30	62	8	0	100	50

breast-feeds a child?" Specifically, we are wondering if membership in La Leche League "causes" women to breast-feed for a longer time than if they were nonmembers. In order to use the table as a tool for determining whether or not one variable is causally influencing another, the percentage of individuals in each of the categories of the independent variable is compared with the percentage of those who fall into a given category of the dependent variable. For example, looking at the 0–5-month category of the dependent variable, we see that 7 percent of the members and 30 percent of the nonmembers fall into this category. In contrast, looking at the 18–23-month category of the dependent variable, we observe that while over one-third (35%) of the members fall into this category, none of the nonmembers do so. In general the table supports the conclusion that membership in the organization does influence how long a woman breast-feeds, with organization members breast-feeding their children for a longer time span than nonmembers.

Notice that, in describing the relationship between the two variables, one moves down the columns of the table. Percentaging of the categories of the independent variable has been done across the rows of the table. A useful rule of thumb to follow in interpreting cross-classification tables of this type is that percentaging is done in one direction and comparisons are made in the other. In order words, if the categories of the independent variable have been percentaged across the rows, interpretive comparisons should be made down the columns. If percentaging has taken place down the columns, then comparisons should be made across the rows.

By presenting data in a tabular form that facilitates comparison the investigator highlights the meaning and importance of data that do not necessarily speak for themselves. It is important to remember, however, that the informed consumer of research need not and should not be entirely dependent on the researcher to interpret the data. By knowing how to read and construct tables you can not only evaluate the investigator's presentation but make your own independent interpretations of the material, which may be different from those of the investigator. Moreover it is sometimes even possible to extend the scope of the author's analysis by making your own comparisons to other data presented in other studies of a same or similar problem.

References

Knafl, K. A. Conflicting perspectives in breast feeding and its management. *American Journal of Nursing* 74:1848, 1974.

Knafl, K.A. Negotiating hospital care: La Leche League members and hospital personnel. *Journal of Obstetric, Gynecologic, and Neonatal Nursing* 5:47, 1976.

43   Meara, H.   La Leche League in the United States: A key to successful
         breast-feeding in a non-supportive culture. *Journal of Nurse Mid-
         wifery* 1:20, 1976.

WORKING WITH AND INTERPRETING DATA

1. In a study entitled "Nursing Intervention with the Presurgical Patient—The Effects of Structured and Unstructured Preoperative Teaching" (*Nursing Research*, July-
   August, 1971) Lindeman and Van Aernam collected data
   from subjects undergoing the following procedures.

   Thyroidectomy
   Pelvic laparotomy
   Cholecystectomy
   Vaginal hysterectomy
   Dilatation and curettage
   Transurethral resection
   Hemorrhoidectomy
   Simple neck dissection
   Radical neck dissection
   Excision of tumor from breast wall
   Inguinal herniorrhaphy
   Thoracotomy
   Appendectomy
   Abdominal hysterectomy
   Gastric resection
   Gastrostomy
   Vaginal tubal ligation
   Cystogram
   Incision and drainage of rectal abscess
   Breast biopsy
   Oophorectomy
   Aneurysm
   Ventral herniorrhaphy
   Pneumonectomy
   Abdominal tubal ligation
   Exploratory laparotomy
   Sympathectomy
   Splenectomy
   Hiatus herniorrhaphy
   Vena cava plication
   Pyloroplasty
   Pyelogram
   Vagotomy
   Bowel resection
   Abdominal perineal resection

Going only by this list, group these data into categories and present them in tabular form. Then look at the article by Lindeman and Van Aernam and compare your categories with theirs. Evaluate the advantages and disadvantages of each categorization scheme.

2. The following data are taken from the study by Knafl and Meara (Knafl, 1974, 1976; Meara, 1976). They indicate when a subsample of 60 La Leche League members first introduced solid foods into the diet of their first child. The plus and minus signs indicate whether or not they were members of the organization at the time of starting their first baby on solids. For each group (member and nonmember) do the following:

   a. Construct a grouped frequency distribution from the data on when solid foods were first introduced. Summarize the nature or pattern of this distribution for each group and compare the two.
   b. What are the true limits and rounded limits of each of your class intervals? Justify your choice of class intervals.
   c. Convert your grouped frequency distributions into percentage distributions.
   d. Convert your grouped frequency distributions into cumulative frequency distributions.
   e. Construct a cross-classification table that indicates when the 60 subjects introduced solid foods and whether they were members of La Leche League at that time. What is the independent variable in the table; what is the dependent variable? Briefly describe the relationship between La Leche League membership and introduction of solid foods as shown in your table.

Data for answering question 2

1. 1 mo +	13. 2 wk −	25. 2 wk −
2. 2 wk −	14. 3 wk −	26. 3 mo +
3. 5 mo −	15. 4 wk −	27. 5 mo +
4. birth −	16. 5 mo +	28. 2 wk −
5. 3 mo −	17. 8 wk −	29. 5 mo +
6. 3 mo +	18. Immediately −	30. 3 wk −
7. 6 mo +	19. 3 wk −	31. 4 wk −
8. 3 mo +	20. 2 mo +	32. 1 mo +
9. 4 mo +	21. 6 mo +	33. 7 wk +
10. 5½ mo +	22. 3 wk −	34. 2½ mo −
11. 6 mo +	23. 2 mo −	35. 1 mo −
12. 6 mo +	24. 1 mo −	36. 6 mo +

37.	2 mo +	45.	1 mo −	53.	1 mo −
38.	4½ mo +	46.	2 wk −	54.	6 wk −
39.	8 wk +	47.	7 wk −	55.	2 wk −
40.	1 mo +	48.	2 wk −	56.	5 mo +
41.	1 mo −	49.	6 mo +	57.	3 mo +
42.	1 mo +	50.	4 wk −	58.	5½ mo +
43.	6 wk −	51.	4 wk +	59.	2 mo +
44.	6 mo +	52.	2 wk −	60.	3 mo +

3. Chaska, Norma L. Status consistency and nurses' expectations and perceptions of role performance. *Nursing Research* 27:356, 1978.
Without referring to the text of the article, describe the frequency distributions presented in Tables 1–3. Compare your interpretation with that of the author.

4. Hampe, Sandra O. Needs of the grieving spouse in a hospital setting. *Nursing Research* 24:113, 1975.
Further summarize and describe the data presented in Table 1 of this article.

5. Elder, Ruth G. Orientation of senior nursing students toward access to contraceptives. *Nursing Research* 25:338, 1976.
Describe the cumulative percentage distributions the author presents in Table 2. Compare the distribution for girls to that for boys.

6. Kayser, Janice Schmit, and Minnigerode, Fred A. Increasing nursing students' interest in working with aged patients. *Nursing Research* 24:23, 1975.
Interpret the cross-classifications presented in Tables 1 and 2 of this article. For each table, what is the authors' dependent and independent variable?

7. Evaluate each author's use of each of the techniques discussed in questions 3–6. Is the technique an appropriate one in terms of the data and the author's purpose? Has the table been constructed so that it promotes communication between the author and the audience?

Graphic Presentation of Data

4

The tables discussed in the previous chapter can all be converted to graphic representations. Since graphs make the pattern of a particular distribution visible, they can be more effective than tables in communicating the meaning of data. Graphs are derived from tables, and like tables they are constructed according to a set of fairly standardized guidelines. Such guidelines give direction to the researcher and facilitate communication by assuring that both researcher and reader are operating under the same general principles.

In this chapter, as in the last, we will consider techniques for summarizing and depicting qualitative as well as quantitative data. Specifically, we will discuss the bar chart and pie chart, which are ways to present qualitative data graphically. We will also discuss the histogram, frequency polygon, and cumulative frequency graph, techniques used to depict quantitative data. Finally, we will discuss the sliding bar chart, a technique for converting two-variable tables into a graphic form.

Graphing Qualitative Data

By using a bar chart the researcher can graphically portray qualitative data, data that cannot be divided into numerical class intervals. In the La Leche League study the investigators asked respondents to specify their method of birth control. How these data were categorized was described in Chapter 3, where they were presented in Table 3.1. Figure 4.1 depicts the same data as a bar chart. This simple-to-construct and easily interpretable graphic form consists of a series of evenly spaced bars of equal widths whose lengths represent category frequencies or proportions. The frequency dimension of the bar chart is usually, but not always, marked off along the *horizontal* axis and the categories of data are marked off along the *vertical* axis. This arrangement makes it possible to label the category represented next to each bar in an easy-to-read manner. While the length of each bar is determined by the number of cases in the category, the width and ordering of the bars is largely a matter of individual discretion. In Figure 4.1 the bars have been arranged from longest to shortest, thereby ordering the class categories by the number of cases falling in them. The bars are of equal width to maximize the neatness and visual appeal of the graph, and they are separated by a space equal in width to half a bar. Since the data are nominal, bars of equal width most accurately reflect the fact that categories cannot be differentiated by a size factor. Bars of unequal width would be misleading, because they would give the impression that the categories were of

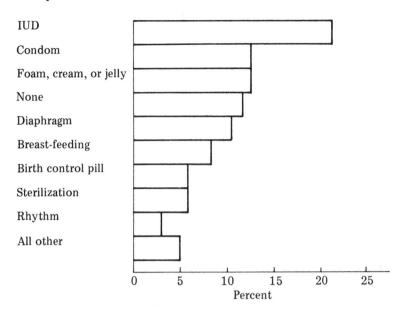

IUD

Condom

Foam, cream, or jelly

None

Diaphragm

Breast-feeding

Birth control pill

Sterilization

Rhythm

All other

0   5   10   15   20   25
Percent

Figure 4.1. Bar chart: Method of birth control for entire sample of La Leche League members. Figure is based on data from 857 subjects and excludes 55 members (6%) who were pregnant when questionnaire was answered.

different sizes. Space between bars emphasizes that the data fall into discrete categories and *not* continuous class intervals. These conventions guide the construction of a precise, easily interpretable graph.

The same data could also have been depicted as a *pie chart* (Fig. 4.2). The circular pie chart is divided into segments or slices. The size of each segment represents the proportion of observations falling into that category. Bar charts and pie charts are equivalent forms for communicating the distribution of data across a series of categories. The choice of one or the other is entirely a matter of personal preference, although the bar chart is more frequently encountered in the professional literature.

Histogram

Figure 4.3 is an example of a histogram. The histogram, which resembles a bar chart turned on its side, is used to depict interval level data. It presents the same information as Table 3.5 in Chapter 3, but in graphic form. It is a graphic equivalent of the grouped frequency distribution. The histogram comprises a series of columns, each column representing one class interval. The height of each column corresponds to the number or percentage of cases in each class. The width of the column is determined by the size of the class intervals. All the columns in Figure 4.3 are of equal

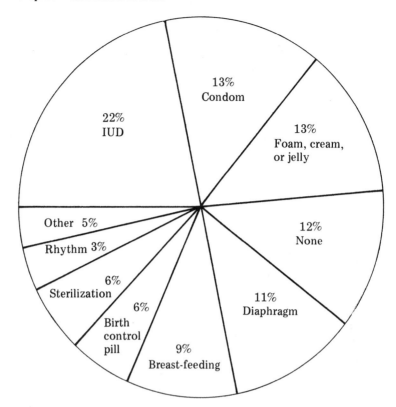

Figure 4.2. Pie chart: Method of birth control for entire sample of La Leche League members. Figure is based on data from 857 subjects and excludes 55 members (6%) who were pregnant at the time questionnaire was answered.

width, since all correspond to a class interval of 6 months. The bars in Figure 4.4 are also all of the same width but represent a class interval of 2 months. The heights of the bars of a histogram vary considerably, since there is a wide variation in the number of cases falling into the various class intervals.

Histograms are constructed with the frequency dimension represented along the *vertical* axis and the class intervals plotted along the *horizontal* axis. The vertical axis should be labeled: frequency, number of subjects or cases, and so forth. The horizontal axis should indicate what the class intervals represent. In the examples, the columns of the histogram have been plotted over the *true* class limits of the class intervals. This is appropriate, since the bars share a common boundary and true class limits represent common boundaries between classes. While it is preferable to demarcate true class limits along the horizontal axis, researchers do not always do this. In all likelihood you will encounter histograms whose columns have been plotted over rounded class limits and class midpoints. Such adaptations of the ideal are usually done to

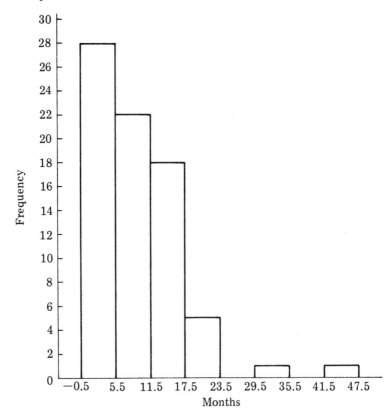

Figure 4.3. Histogram: Duration of first breast-feeding experience for a subsample of La Leche League members.

streamline the graph by decreasing the number of figures along the horizontal axis. In constructing a histogram, it is customary to leave a space between the vertical axis and the first bar as has been done in Figures 4.3 and 4.4 to improve readability.

While the intervals along the horizontal scale may or may not begin with zero, the frequency axis *must* originate with zero. Investigators who do not conform to this principle present a distorted view of the distribution of their cases. Figure 4.5 illustrates why this is the case. Note that the ratio between the number of cases in the first two categories is 20 to 30 or 2:3. This is pictorially conveyed when the frequency axis begins at zero, since the height of the second column is 1½ times the first. Similarly, the third interval contains twice as many cases as the first and the third column is twice the height of the first. When the frequency axis does not originate with zero, however, the graph no longer visually represents the comparative proportion of cases in each category. When the frequency axis begins at 10, it makes it look as if the second interval contains twice as many cases as the first and the third contains three times as many cases as the first, which

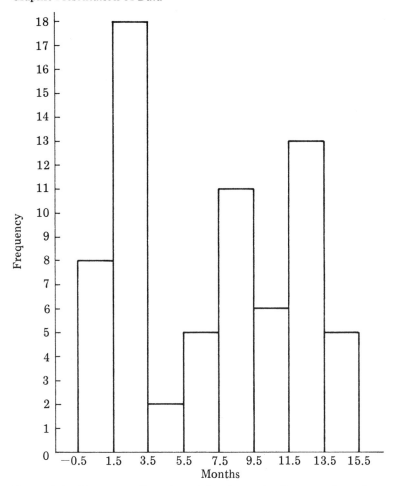

Figure 4.4. Histogram: Duration of first breast-feeding experience for a subsample of 75 La Leche League members.

they do not. Failure to begin the frequency axis at zero distorts or clouds the meaning of the data. As a critical consumer, you should be aware of such violations of the principles of graphing data.

Investigators can also give varying impressions of the nature of their data by manipulating the lengths of the horizontal and vertical axes. Although Figures 4.6 and 4.7 depict the same data as Figure 4.3, the impression they convey as to the nature of the distribution of cases is different. By elongating the horizontal axis, as in Figure 4.6, the researcher makes it look *as if* the data are distributed over a wide range of values. At first glance the figure is likely to communicate the message that the data are widely varied. Figure 4.7, in which the horizontal axis is shortened relative to the vertical, conveys the opposite impression, although it depicts the same set of data. By keeping the two axes of a histogram *approximately* the same length, the researcher reduces the possibility that his or her

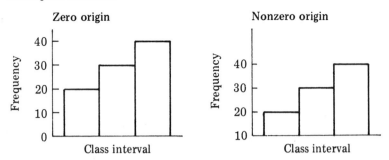

Figure 4.5. Histograms with zero and nonzero origins of frequency axes.

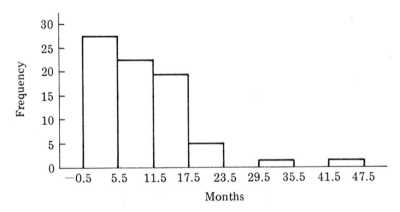

Figure 4.6. Histogram: Duration of first breast-feeding experience for a subsample of La Leche League members.

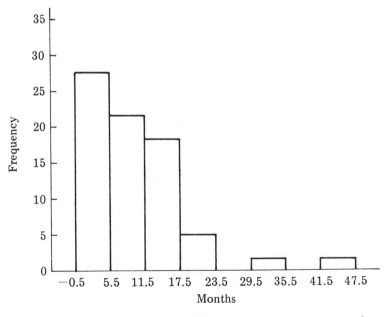

Figure 4.7. Histogram: Duration of first breast-feeding experience for a subsample of La Leche League members.

graph will be misleading. However, it is not a hard and fast rule that the axes of a graph be of equal length. Therefore the reader should carefully inspect any graph before drawing conclusions about the nature of the distribution being portrayed.

A special problem arises if we want to convert a grouped frequency distribution having *unequal* class intervals into a histogram. For example, the last category in the following distribution is three times the width of the others, 18 as opposed to six months.

Class interval	f
0– 5	28
6–11	22
12–17	18
18–35	6
	$N = 74$

The most obvious way to handle this situation graphically might be to make the column representing the last category three times the width of the columns representing the other class intervals. This solution to depicting unequal class intervals is shown in Figure 4.8.

The solution in Figure 4.8 is unsatisfactory, however, because it gives a misleading impression of the data. It is misleading because, although there are only six observations in the entire 17.5–35.5 class, the area within the corresponding histogram column is the same as the area allocated to the 18 observations in the 11.5–17.5 class interval. In other words, when we increase the width of the class interval without making any adjustment in the height of the bar, we no longer visually represent the comparative proportion of cases in each category. Pictorially it looks as if the last two categories have the same number of cases. In actuality the last class interval has only *one-third* as many observations as the category preceding it. In sum, Figure 4.8 allocates three times more area to the final class interval than it merits.

The usual approach to graphing unequal class intervals is shown in Figure 4.9. In this graph an adjustment has been made in the height of the final bar to compensate for its greater width. Since the width is three times that of the other bars, we have divided the frequency by 3 in order to arrive at an adjusted frequency that accurately represents the proportion of cases in the class interval. In effect we are treating the 17.5–35.5 class interval *as if* it were *three* categories, each of which is of equal width (6 units) with the other categories in the distributions. Moreover we are assuming that the six observations in the 17.5–35.5 category are evenly distributed across this class interval, with two observations every 6 units

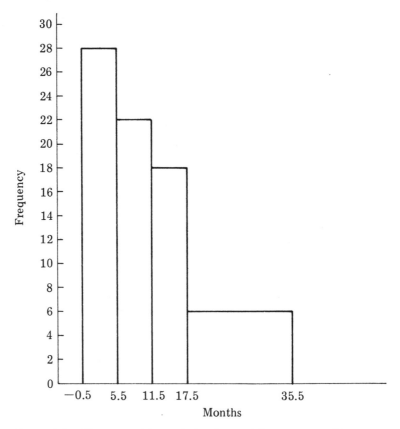

Figure 4.8. Histogram: Unequal class interval (incorrect graphing technique).

or months. Accordingly we have depicted the data as if there are two observations each between 18 and 23 months, 24 and 29 months, and 30 and 35 months.

When the assumption of even distribution of cases across class intervals is inaccurate, the technique employed in Figure 4.9 will misrepresent the data. Referring back to Table 3.5 from which this example was derived, we see that five observations fell into the 18–23 category, *zero* observations fell into the 24–29 category, and one observation fell into the 30–35 category. Since Figure 4.9 makes it look as if two cases fell into each of these intervals, it does somewhat misrepresent the data. However, it misrepresents the data less than does Figure 4.8, which makes it look as if there are 18 observations in a category that in fact contains only 6. In short, Figure 4.9 is the lesser of two evils. It is an acceptable, but not wholly satisfactory, solution to the problem of unequal class intervals.

The most satisfactory solution to the problem is to avoid it altogether by casting data in equally sized intervals. If, because of the nature of the data, this is not appropriate,

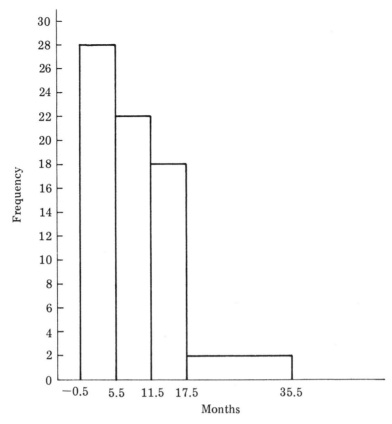

Figure 4.9. Histogram: Unequal class interval (correct graphing technique).

then any unequal interval should be converted into a multiple of the other intervals in size, e.g., twice or three times the width of the others. When unequal intervals are represented in this way, it is then a relatively simple procedure to adjust the height of the bar when drawing a histogram. To review, this is done by dividing the frequency of the unequal class interval by however many times the unequal interval exceeds the other intervals in size. For example, if one class interval is twice as large as the others, and that interval contains ten cases, the corresponding bar on a histogram would be twice the width of the others, but the frequency would be adjusted so that the height of the bar would be equivalent to 5 (10 divided by 2) and not 10.

When one class interval is smaller than the rest, the reverse of the above procedure can be followed. The unequal interval can be depicted as one-half or one-third the width of the others. In this case, however, the height of the bar is adjusted by *multiplying* the number of observations in the interval by however many times smaller that interval is than the others.

Finally, if there are open class intervals, it is not possible to convert a grouped frequency distribution into a histogram unless the open interval(s) are arbitrarily closed.

While the above procedures provide acceptable techniques for dealing with the problem of graphing class categories of unequal sizes, it is a problem that is usually easy to avoid altogether. Given that unequal class intervals complicate the process of constructing a graph and may, from the reader's viewpoint, lead to a somewhat confusing presentation of the data, the best course of action is to create class intervals of equal size at the outset of the data analysis.

Taking into account the various concepts and principles touched on in this discussion, we can summarize the procedures for drawing a histogram as follows:

1. Construct a vertical axis and a horizontal axis of approximately equal lengths.
2. Mark off class intervals along the horizontal axis, using *true* class limits.
3. Whenever possible, maintain class intervals of equal width.
4. Mark off the number or percentage of cases in each class along the vertical axis.
5. Originate the vertical axis at zero.
6. Clearly label both axes and clearly and completely title the entire graph.

Having described the techniques for constructing a histogram, we can now turn our attention to interpreting the data we have so carefully depicted.

We have spoken throughout this section about the nature or shape of a distribution of observations. Researchers draw on a standard vocabulary to characterize the distribution of their data. Often they refer to cases as being either positively or negatively *skewed*. A skewed distribution has a few extreme cases at one end of it. Figure 4.3 could be described as being skewed positively, since there are extreme cases at the high, or positive, end of the distribution. Had the extreme cases fallen at the low end of the distribution, it would have been described as negatively skewed. Figure 4.10 shows the general shape of positively and negatively skewed distributions. A distribution with a few extreme or outlying cases in the upper or right-hand tail of the curve is described as positively skewed; one with a few cases in the left-hand tail of the curve is negatively skewed. Not all distributions are skewed, and those that are not are generally described as symmetrical. A symmetrical distribution has approximately the same number of extremely high as extremely low scores, such as Figure 4.12.

Investigators also refer to distributions as being peaked or flat. Figure 4.11 illustrates this characteristic of a distribution. Peaked distributions are said to be *leptokurtic*, flat distribu-

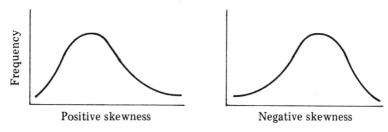

Figure 4.10. General shape of positively and negatively skewed distributions.

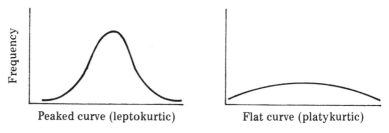

Figure 4.11. General shape of peaked and flat distributions.

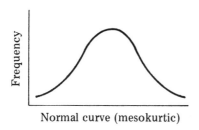

Figure 4.12. Normal (bell) curve.

tions are *platykurtic*, and those that are neither are described as *mesokurtic*. Perhaps the most familiar shape of a distribution is the normal or *bell curve* depicted in Figure 4.12. It is a symmetrical, mesokurtic curve. The normal curve has additional characteristics that make it extremely useful in statistical analysis. These properties will be discussed at length in Chapter 7. Although terms such as *skewness* and *kurtosis* may seem unnecessarily jargonish, they facilitate precise, efficient descriptions of data and thereby aid communication of research findings.

Frequency Polygon

Figure 4.13 presents an alternative form for graphing the data presented in Figure 4.3. Figure 4.13 is an example of a *frequency polygon*, and as Figure 4.14 demonstrates, it is equivalent to and can be derived from a histogram. By connecting the midpoints of the column tops of the histogram with

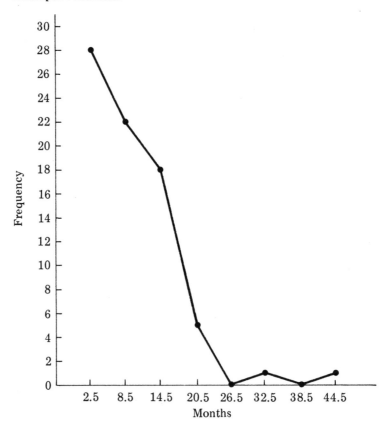

Figure 4.13. Frequency polygon: Duration of first breast-feeding experience for a subsample of 75 La Leche League members.

straight lines, one can superimpose a frequency polygon on a histogram. In practice a researcher would select one or the other of these means of presenting data.

The procedure for constructing a frequency polygon parallels that for constructing a histogram. First, two axes are drawn perpendicular to each other. The vertical axis is used to represent the number or percentage of cases in each class interval and is labeled frequency, number of subjects, cases, and so forth. The horizontal axis represents the class intervals. As in the histogram, these axes should be of *approximately* equal lengths to avoid giving a misleading impression of the data. The vertical axis should originate at zero. On the other hand, although the vertical axis must originate with zero, it is sometimes impractical to represent all values between zero and the value of the first observation along this axis. For example, if one observation ranged in value from 100 to 200, it would unnecessarily elongate the vertical axis to represent all values between zero and 200, since there are no observations between

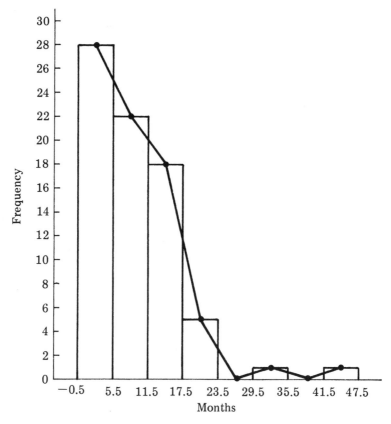

Figure 4.14. Histogram: Superimposed frequency polygon of duration of breast-feeding experience for a subsample of 75 La Leche League members.

zero and 100. In instances such as this it is possible to "interrupt" the vertical axis in the following manner:

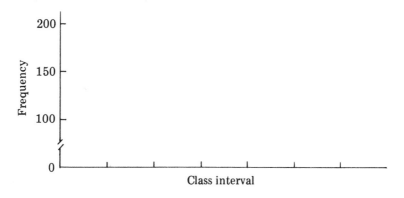

If you do this, or are interpreting a graph that has an "interrupted" vertical axis, it is important to remember that the graph will no longer visually represent the comparative proportion of cases in each category.

In contrast to the histogram, which shows the true class limits along the horizontal axis, the frequency polygon is plotted over the *midpoint* of each class interval. The midpoint of the class interval is the point that divides the interval into two equal sections: the midpoint has one-half the interval above it and one-half the interval below it. When working with data that have been rounded to the nearest unit, one can find the class midpoint by adding together the upper and lower *true* limits of the class and dividing by 2. This procedure is demonstrated with the following class intervals:

Class interval	True class interval	Calculation of class midpoint
0-5	− .5- 5.5	$\dfrac{-.5 + 5.5}{2} = \dfrac{5}{2} = 2.5$
6-11	5.5-11.5	$\dfrac{5.5 + 11.5}{2} = \dfrac{17}{2} = 8.5$
12-17	11.5-17.5	$\dfrac{11.5 + 17.5}{2} = \dfrac{29}{2} = 14.5$

Points are plotted over these midpoints at heights corresponding to the frequency or number of cases in each class. The points are then connected to one another by straight lines.

Researchers sometimes choose to close the ends of a frequency polygon by extending them to the horizontal axis. When this is done, the polygon is connected to the baseline at what would be the midpoint of the next class interval *below* the lowest one and at what would be the midpoint of the next class interval *above* the highest one. Tying the frequency polygon to the horizontal baseline is largely a matter of personal choice and is not done by all researchers.

Since histograms and frequency polygons are equivalent graphic forms, you may be wondering if an understanding of both is really necessary. Of course from a consumer standpoint it is, since both kinds of graphs are found in the literature. In addition there are times when the frequency polygon is the more appropriate form to use. This is the case when the researcher wants to superimpose two or more distributions on the same pair of axes for comparative purposes. Figure 4.15 depicts the length of breast-feeding experience for the subsample of 75 La Leche League members and for another, hypothetical, sample of 75 nonmembers. (If we were comparing samples of unequal size, then it would be necessary to represent percentages and not raw numbers along the vertical axis.)

Comparing the two distributions we can see that the one for members is more spread out than the one for nonmem-

Graphic Presentation of Data

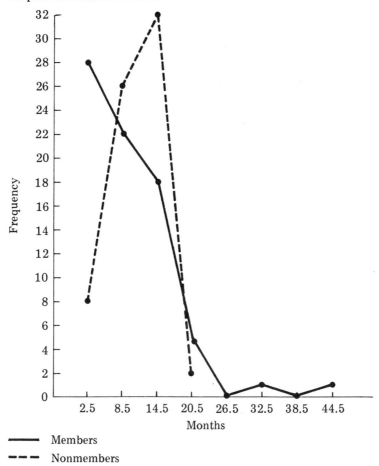

Figure 4.15. Frequency polygon: Comparative length of first completed breast-feeding experience for La Leche League members and nonmembers.

bers. Whereas the members' breast-feeding experiences last from between 2.5 and 44.5 months, the nonmembers' experiences range from 2.5 to 20.5 months. On the other hand, while more of the members fell more frequently into the 2.5-month category than into any other category, nonmembers were most likely to fall into the 14.5-month category. Comparisons such as these are made visible when data from two or more samples are depicted on the same frequency polygon.

Because they have fewer overlapping lines, superimposed frequency polygons are easier to interpret than superimposed histograms would be. Another advantage to the frequency polygon is that it provides a closer approximation to a smooth curve than the histogram does. We usually describe and interpret these graphs with reference to a particular kind of curve (skewed, peaked), and the frequency polygon makes the relationship between the distribution and a specific curve more apparent. Moreover the frequency polygon can accommodate unequal class intervals without special adjustments or manipulations of the data.

The basic precepts governing the construction of a frequency polygon can be summarized as follows:

1. Construct a vertical and a horizontal axis of approximately equal lengths.
2. Mark off class intervals along the horizontal axis, using class midpoints.
3. Mark off the number or percentage of cases in each class along the vertical axis.
4. Originate the vertical axis at zero.
5. Clearly label both axes and clearly and completely title the entire graph.

Cumulative Frequency Graph

Like the cumulative frequency table, cumulative frequency graphs deal with the percentage of cases above or below a certain point in a distribution. Figures 4.16 and 4.17 are examples of more-than and less-than cumulative graphs. As in these examples, the more-than graph always runs from the upper left corner to the lower right corner of the graph; the less-than graph always originates in the lower left corner and extends to the upper right corner. Cumulative frequency graphs are also called *ogives*. The construction of a cumulative

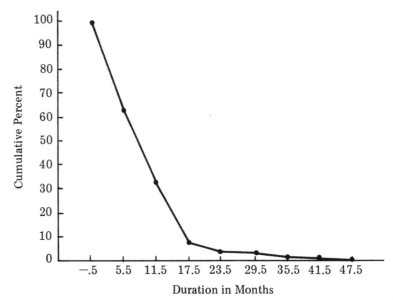

Figure 4.16. More-than cumulative graph: Duration of first completed breast-feeding experience for a subsample of 75 La Leche League members.

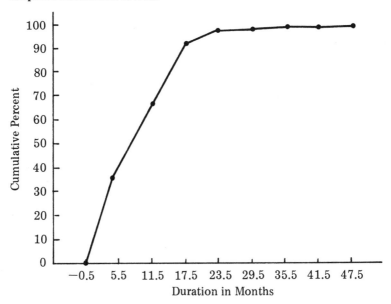

Figure 4.17. Less-than cumulative graph: Duration of first completed breast-feeding experience for a subsample of 75 La Leche League members.

graph begins as with other graphs, with plotting two axes, a vertical axis to express frequency and a horizontal axis to depict class intervals. A slight variation from this standard procedure is that in the cumulative graph the frequencies along the vertical axis are expressed in terms of a cumulative percentage. Accordingly this axis is labeled from 0 to 100 percent. Cumulative frequency graphs are plotted over true class limits. Specifically, a "more-than" graph is plotted over the true *lower* limits of each class interval and a "less-than" graph is plotted over the true *upper* limits of each class interval. Figures 4.16 and 4.17 portray the data presented in Tables 3.9 and 3.10. As for all graphs the construction of a specific cumulative frequency graph is undertaken only after the corresponding table of data has been formulated.

The true class intervals for the data depicted in Figures 4.16 and 4.17 are

−0.5- 5.5
5.5-11.5
11.5-17.5
17.5-23.5
23.5-29.5
29.5-35.5
35.5-41.5
41.5-47.5

To construct the more-than graph we begin by plotting the percentage of women who breast-fed for more than − 0.5

months, the *lower* true class limit of the first class interval. We continue by plotting the percentage of women breast-feeding for more than 5.5, 11.5, 17.5, 23.5, 29.5, 35.5, and 41.5 months. To construct the less-than graph we begin by plotting the percentage of women breast-feeding for less than 5.5 months, the *upper* true class limit of the first class interval. We then plot the percentage of women breast-feeding for less than 11.5, 17.5, 23.5, 29.5, 35.5, 41.5, and 47.5 months, the remaining true upper limits of the class intervals. In both graphs, once these points have been plotted, they are connected by straight lines. Although working from a different reference point, the two graphs present the same data. A researcher would thus use either a more-than or a less-than graph but not both. While not mandatory, the researcher may "tie" or connect the graph line to the horizontal axis of the graph.

Cumulative graphs not only describe a distribution but allow the reader to make certain interpretations of the data. For descriptive purposes the cumulative graph depicts the rate at which cases are cumulating into successive categories. Figure 4.18 illustrates some shapes frequently encountered in

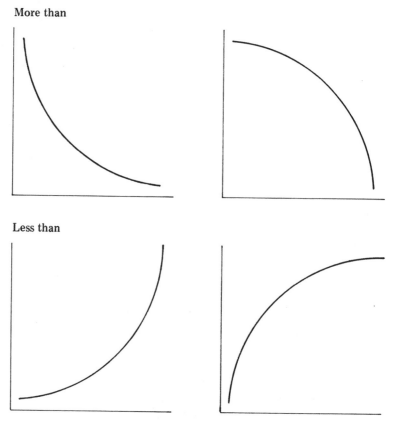

Figure 4.18. Typical shapes of cumulative frequency graphs.

cumulative frequency graphs. The distributions shown in this figure are: (a) decreasing at a decreasing rate, (b) decreasing at an increasing rate, (c) increasing at an increasing rate, and (d) increasing at a decreasing rate.

With regard to interpreting the data, we might like to know the percentage of people who breast-fed for more than 5 months. To determine this, we locate approximately where 5 months would fall on the horizontal scale in Figure 4.16. We then extend a perpendicular line from the baseline to the cumulative frequency curve. From the point at which this line and the curve intersect, we draw a second line, parallel to the baseline. The point at which this second line intersects the vertical axis tells us the percentage of women who breast-fed more than 5 months (approximately 60 percent). By following this procedure we can determine the percentage of respondents falling above or below *any* point in the distribution, regardless of whether or not it corresponds to an actual observation.

These cumulative graphs can also be used to ascertain a value below or above which a certain percentage of the cases fall. For example, we can use a cumulative graph to find the median of a distribution, the point that divides the distribution in half. The process is the reverse of that just described. Starting this time at the vertical axis, we extend a line parallel to the horizontal axis from the 50 percent mark to the curve, and then drop a perpendicular line from the curve to the baseline. The point of intersection in this instance tells us that approximately 50 percent of the subjects breast-fed for more than 8 months and 50 percent breast-fed for less than 8 months. Using this technique we can find the number of months corresponding to any percentage on the frequency scale. Because cumulative graphs facilitate interpretation of the data, they are highly useful graphic techniques. Figure 4.19 illustrates the use of a cumulative frequency graph for the purposes discussed above.

Graphing Two Variables

By constructing a *sliding bar chart* it is possible to depict cross-classifications in graphic form. Figure 4.20 exemplifies this technique. The sliding bar chart is an effective way to highlight visually the difference between or among a number of different groups. Figure 4.20 presents the same data as Table 3.13, although the data on duration of the breast-feeding experience have been collapsed into two categories. In this kind of chart there are as many bars as there are groups being compared. A vertical axis cuts across each bar and acts as a boundary between categories. Bars are of equal size and are arranged on the vertical axis according to the proportion of the observations in the group that fall into

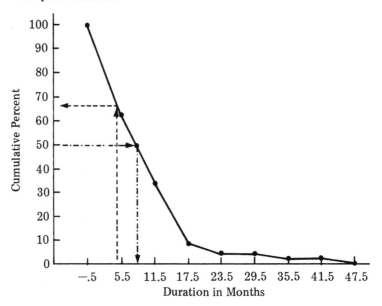

Figure 4.19. Use of a cumulative frequency graph for interpretive purposes.

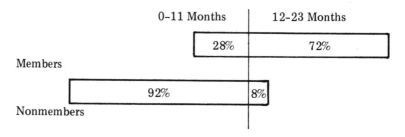

	0–11 Months	12–23 Months
Members	28%	72%
Nonmembers	92%	8%

Figure 4.20. Sliding bar chart: Duration of first breast-feeding experience for 75 members of La Leche League and 75 nonmembers.

each of the two categories. Each bar represents 100 percent of the observations in the group just as in Table 3.13, where percentages were based on the total number of cases in each row. The purpose of the sliding bar chart is to make group differences visually apparent. As Figure 4.20 illustrates, most of the bar representing members falls to the right of the perpendicular axis; most of the bar representing nonmembers falls to the left of this axis. The greater the alignment between or among bars, the greater the similarity between or among groups. Conversely, decreasing alignments indicate increasing differences between or among groups.

The guidelines given in Chapter 3 for interpreting and evaluating tables also apply to graphs and charts. Graphs and charts should be clearly labeled and contain sufficient information to stand alone—that is, be understandable without reference to the text of a specific book or article in which they are presented. On the other hand the author should discuss the graphic material in the body of his or her text, highlighting what he or she identifies as important points. As a reader you should critically consider the quality of both the graphic presentation and the discussion. In so doing you compare your own understanding and interpretation of the material to that of the authors. As you develop your skills as a critical consumer of research literature, you are likely to find yourself more willing and able to expand and sometimes even challenge the interpretations and presentations made by others.

WORKING WITH AND INTERPRETING DATA

1. Use the data presented in question 1 of Chapter 3 to construct a bar chart.

2. Use the data presented in question 2 of Chapter 3 to construct the following for both member and nonmember groups:

   a. A histogram *or* a frequency polygon.
   b. A more-than *or* a less-than cumulative frequency graph (ogive).

3. Describe in words the nature or pattern of the distribution as depicted in the graphs you have constructed in questions 1 and 2.

4. The authors of the following articles present data in graphic form. For each article, describe the findings presented in graphs and evaluate the author's use of this descriptive technique.

   Brock, Leah. Automobile transportation in community health services. *Nursing Outlook* 23:378, 1975.
   Freihofer, Patricia, and Geraldene Felton. Nursing behaviors in bereavement: An exploratory study. *Nursing Research* 25:332, 1976.
   Kerpelman, Larry C. Films in nursing education. *Nursing Outlook* 23:35, 1975.
   Ward, John A., and John M. Griffen. Improving instruction through computer-graded examinations. *Nursing Outlook* 25:524, 1977.
   Williams, Karen R., and Barbara C. Walike. Effect of the temperature of tube feeding on gastric motility in monkeys. *Nursing Research* 24:4, 1975.

Measures of Central Tendency and Location

Chapters 3 and 4 discuss various methods for grouping observations together and presenting them in a table or graph so that the total set of data may be described and summarized. Although they communicate a great deal of valuable information, these methods have two major limitations. First, they tend to be somewhat cumbersome and uneconomical ways to summarize a data set, and second, they are dead end approaches that cannot be used directly in any further statistical analysis of the data. This chapter will discuss various methods of summarizing an entire set of data by reporting a *single* characteristic or value that can be used to describe the general nature of the distribution of observations within the data set.

These summary characteristics or values are generally referred to as measures of *central tendency* and measures of *location*. Specifically, the measures that will be discussed in this chapter are the mode, the median, the mean, and quantiles. Each of these measures provides a unique kind of summary description of a set of data. Of them, the mean is especially important, because it is included in computations for many of the more advanced analytical techniques.

Measures of central tendency are commonly referred to as *averages* because they represent a kind of norm around which observed values tend to vary. As the name implies, measures of central tendency may be thought of in a very loose sense as telling us where the middle of a distribution is located. It is important to bear in mind, however, that measures of central tendency are not necessarily identical with the exact center of a set of data. Instead they represent a functional center of a distribution, in that they tell us that most of the observations *tend* to be located at or near a particular point. For example, the mode is the most frequently occurring observation in a distribution; the median is the point in an array of ordinal or interval level observations that divides the array into two equal parts, and thus represents the "visual center" of a distribution; the mean is the arithmetic average of all the values in a distribution of interval level observations, and thus represents the "central value" of a distribution.

Mode

The most frequently occurring observation or value in a distribution is called the *mode*. Thus the mode tells us the category or value where the concentration of observations is the greatest.

Computation

The mode is easily calculated when working with nominal data such as that presented in Table 5.1. Most of the respondents

Table 5.1. Obtaining the Mode for a Nominal Level Variable: Usual Source of Medical Care

Usual source of care	f	
Doctor's office	316	Mode = Doctor's office
Hospital outpatient clinic	62	
Other clinic	22	
Hospital emergency room	21	
Doctor's office and hospital emergency room	31	
Other combined sources	30	
Other	27	
No usual place	6	
Total	515	
(No answer = 2)		

to the questionnaire on which this table is based reported a doctor's office as their usual source of medical care. Therefore the mode is "doctor's office." Note that the mode is *not* the value 316, which is simply the frequency count of the observations that occur in the modal category.

When dealing with interval level data as in Table 5.2, the mode is identified as the class interval with the highest frequency. Thus the modal distance to their usual source of medical care among these respondents is 0–9 miles. But rather than expressing the mode in terms of the range of values that are included in the modal category, researchers often prefer to express the mode simply as a single value which may be considered representative of all the values included in

Table 5.2. Obtaining the Mode for an Interval Level Variable: Distance to Usual Source of Medical Care

Distance (miles)*	f	
0–9	232	Mode = 0–9 or 4.5 miles
10–19	204	
20–29	63	
30–39	7	
40–49	1	
50–59	1	
Total	508	
(No usual source = 6)		
(Don't know = 1)		
(No answer = 2)		

*Rounded to nearest whole mile.

the modal class interval. Since the data in Table 5.2 are in grouped form, we do not know how the 232 observations in the modal category are distributed across the range of values from 0 to 9 miles. If we assume that the observations are distributed *evenly* across the class interval, our best choice of a representative value is the midpoint of the modal class interval, because in most cases the midpoint will be centrally located among the observations in the interval. Accordingly the mode for the data presented in Table 5.2 would be reported as 4.5 miles.

To report the mode for Table 5.2 as either 0–9 or 4.5 would be somewhat misleading, however, since it would not reflect the presence of an almost equally strong concentration of observations in the 10–19 interval, which contains 204 cases. Although it runs contrary to our purpose of deriving a single value to summarize the central tendency of a distribution, in situations such as this the researcher may decide that a more useful summary of the data would be provided if the distribution were described as *bimodal*. Thus two modes would be reported, one having a value of 4.5 and the other a value of 14.5. Note that it is not necessary that the two categories with the highest frequencies contain an equal number of observations for a distribution to be considered bimodal. The decision regarding whether the number of observations in another interval is sufficiently large to be considered as a second mode is left to the judgment of the researcher.

An alternative strategy in the situation in Table 5.2, in which an overwhelming majority of the observations are distributed almost equally across two adjacent class intervals, is to regroup the data so as to merge the two modal categories into one. Thus the regrouped distribution presented in Table 5.3 has only one mode, which is located in the 0–19 interval and may be expressed as the value 9.5, the class midpoint. It should be noted, however, that while regrouping has elimin-

Table 5.3. Obtaining the Mode for an Interval Level Variable: Distance to Usual Source of Medical Care, Regrouped

Distance (miles)*	f	
0–19	436	Mode = 0–19 or 9.5 miles
20–39	70	
40–59	2	
Total	508	
(No usual source = 6)		
(Don't know = 1)		
(No answer = 2)		

*Rounded to nearest whole mile.

ated the problem of bimodality, it has meant a sacrifice of some precision in the summary of the data. The mode of 9.5 is a compromise between the competing values of 4.5 and 14.5 and does not reflect the fact that the observations are actually distributed in two clusters, one centered around 4.5 and one around 14.5. Also, considering that if a single mode were reported for Table 5.2, that mode would be 4.5, the regrouping of the data in Table 5.3 has caused a considerable shift in the modal value up to 9.5, which is more than twice as large. The decision as to which strategy to employ will depend upon the researcher's purpose in analyzing the data. If a single and general description of the data is desired, then regrouping is more efficient than reporting two modes, which is usually done when a more thorough and precise description is needed.

Of course, it is not feasible to eliminate bimodality by regrouping if the two modes are separated by several class intervals rather than being located in adjacent intervals. For example, one mode might have been located in the 0–9 interval and the other in the 50–59 interval, indicating that people travel either relatively short or relatively long distances, with few traveling in the 10–49 mile range. In that case, in order to merge the two modal intervals, the researcher would have to condense the entire distribution into one huge class interval of 0–59. Such a radical regrouping of the data would communicate very little information about the nature of the distribution. Instead the best procedure would be to report the two modes of 4.5 and 54.5.

When computing the mode for a set of grouped data, the scope of the categories, or the width of the class intervals, must be equal to avoid a misrepresentation of the data. For example, Table 5.4 is generated by regrouping the data pre-

Table 5.4. Obtaining the Mode for an Interval Level Variable: Distance to Usual Source of Medical Care, Regrouped

Distance (miles)*	f	
0–9	232	
10–29	267	Mode = 10–29 or 19.5 miles
30–39	7	
40–49	1	
50–59	1	
Total	508	
(No usual source = 6)		
(Don't know = 1)		
(No answer = 2)		

*Rounded to nearest whole mile.

sented in Table 5.2 and has a mode equal to 19.5 as compared with the mode of 4.5 for Table 5.2. The mode for Table 5.4 is misleading, because the modal class interval, 10–29 miles, is twice as wide as all the others and thus has a better chance of including a large number of observations since it covers a larger portion of the measurement scale. While the width of class intervals can be calculated precisely for interval level variables, the breadth of nominal level categories is often less obvious. For example, the modal category for Table 5.5 is "physician," since most of the observations are located in that category. However, the scope of that category is much broader than the others, which are dental specialties. If the dental categories are grouped together and placed in a category labeled "dentists," which is similar in scope to the "physician" category, we find that Table 5.5 contains 100 physicians and 100 dentists. Therefore the initial grouping into categories of unequal size was misleading.

Advantages

Perhaps the main advantage to using the mode as opposed to the median or the mean as a measure of central tendency is that the mode is very quick and easy to compute. Once a set of data have been arranged in a frequency distribution, the mode is simply identified by means of a visual inspection of the frequency column. A second advantage of the mode is that it is useful for describing distributions that have more than one point of central tendency because more than one mode may be reported. This may provide a more complete summary of the data than use of the median or the mean, which give only a single value. However, it is usually inefficient to report more than two modes for a distribution. Finally, the mode is especially useful for analyzing nominal level data because, as we will see in the following sections of this chapter, the mode is the only measure of central tendency that can be applied to nominal level data. While the mode may be computed for data at any level of measurement, the median requires either ordinal or interval level measurement, and the mean can be computed only for interval level data.

Table 5.5. Distribution of 200 Health Professionals by Profession

Profession	f
Physician	100
Orthodontist	25
Endodontist	40
Periodontist	35
Total	200

74

Disadvantages

While the possibility of computing more than one mode for some distributions may be viewed as an advantage, it is also a major disadvantage of using the mode as a measure of central tendency. This is because our purpose is to derive a *single* characteristic or value to describe the general nature of all the observations in a data set. Furthermore, although we have looked only at examples of bimodality, it is possible for some distributions to have three or even more modes. The most extreme case of multimodality would occur if every category or class interval in a distribution had exactly the same frequency. One way of looking at this situation is to say that any and every category or interval may be considered as the mode. On the other hand, since no one category or interval stands out from all the rest, this situation is best viewed as one in which there is *no* mode at all.

Bimodality often results from the combination of two distinct populations of observations into a single distribution. For example, the distribution of the weight of a group of female patients might be unimodal, with a mode near 125 pounds, while that for a group of male patients might be unimodal, with a mode near 175 pounds. If these two distributions were merged, a bimodal distribution would be obtained, with modes located near 125 and 175 pounds. It is important for a researcher to remain alert to the possibility that any bimodal distribution may indicate the presence of two distinct populations that should be analyzed separately.

Another disadvantage of the mode is that it is an unstable measure of central tendency. As we observed in Tables 5.2 and 5.3, the value of the mode may fluctuate greatly as a result of different methods of grouping the observations. Furthermore, as we observed in Tables 5.4 and 5.5, the location of the mode is influenced by the scope of the categories or the width of the class intervals. Finally, since the mode is derived by the process of visual inspection rather than by mathematical calculations, even when analyzing interval level data, the mode is rarely useful in further statistical computations.

Median

The *median* is the point that divides an array or frequency distribution into two equal parts such that half the observations are below and half are above that point. The procedure for computing the median differs according to whether the data are ungrouped or grouped.

Computation: Ungrouped Data

Table 5.6 presents arrays of the ages of two groups of terminally ill patients. Let us first consider array A and compute its median.

Table 5.6. Obtaining the Median from an Array of Interval Level Data: Ages of Two Groups of Terminally Ill Patients

Array A (N is odd)	Array B (N is even)
40	40
45	45
48	48
51	51
55	55
56	56
59	59
60	60
64	
$N = 9$	$N = 8$
$\dfrac{N}{2} = \dfrac{9}{2} = 4.5$	$\dfrac{N}{2} = \dfrac{8}{2} = 4$
Median $= 55$	Median $= \dfrac{51 + 55}{2} = \dfrac{106}{2} = 53$

Starting at either end of the array, with the person with the lowest or highest age, the median is computed by *counting off* observations until we arrive at the observation that is located exactly in the center of the array. To locate this observation we must think of each observation as occupying a rank from 1 through N (9 in this case) in the array. The median is the observation that occupies the middle rank, with an equal number of ranks located both below and above it. The median's rank is determined by dividing the total number of observations in the array by 2 and then counting off that number of observations into the array. In this case $N/2 = 9/2 = 4.5$. If we begin with the low end of the array, we count off the observation with a value of 40, then 45, and so on. By the time we count off the observation whose value is 51, we have counted off four observations and have only a one-half count to go. This one-half count means the next observation (55) should be exactly in the center of the array. We find this to be true: observation 55 is located in the center of the array because it has four observations located below and four located above it. Therefore the value of the median in this array is 55, which tells us that one-half the observations have a value of less than 55 and one-half have a value of more than 55.

The computation of the median as the observation that is located in the center of an array is straightforward when the total number of observations (N) is an odd number such as 9 in array A. But an additional step is required to compute the median when N is an even number, as is the case of array B in Table 5.6, which has eight observations. For this array, $N/2 = 8/2 = 4$. Beginning with the low end of the array we count off four observations and discover that the center of the array is located in the interval *between* the observations of 51 and 55. In order to derive a single value to report as the median, the average (mean) of the values that are located on either side of the center point of the array is computed by adding them together and dividing their sum by 2. Thus, the median of array B is computed as: $(51 + 55)/2 = 106/2 = 53$.

Computation: Grouped Data

When an array has been collapsed into a grouped frequency distribution, however, it is not possible to count off individual observations until we reach the center of the distribution, because we do not know the actual value of individual observations. All we know in this case is that each observation has a value within a certain range as indicated by the lower and upper limits of the class interval. For example, let us return to the data regarding distance to usual source of medical care presented in Table 5.2, $N/2 = 508/2 = 254$. Beginning at the low end of the distribution, we count off the 232 observations in the 0–9 interval and then continue into the 10–19 interval until we count off a total of 254 observations. But our dilemma is that we do not know what value corresponds to the 254th case. While we know that it is one of the 204 observations that fall in the 10–19 interval, we do not know precisely where it is located within that range.

Fortunately there is a method of estimating the value of the median for a grouped frequency distribution, and this method serves very well in the majority of cases. In mathematics this method is referred to as *interpolation.* Although the formula for computing an interpolated median is rather formidable in appearance, it is no more than a shorthand set of instructions for a logical process. Therefore we will first discuss this process so as to give you an intuitive understanding of it before introducing the formula.

In order to arrive at an interpolated estimate of the median for a grouped frequency distribution, we must first generate a less-than *cumulated frequency* (*cf*) column, as shown in Table 5.7. Examining the cumulated frequencies we see that we will count off the 254th ($N/2$) observation somewhere in the 10–19 class interval. We also see that by the time we left the 0–9 interval we had counted off 232 observations, leaving 22 ($254 - 232 = 22$) additional observations to be counted off from among the 204 observations that are contained in the 10–19 interval. Since we do not know exactly how these 204 observations are distributed across the range of values from 9.5 to 19.5 (using true limits), we will assume that they are distributed *evenly* across the entire interval, which contains a

Table **5.7**. Obtaining the Median from Grouped Data: Distance to Usual Source of Medical Care

Distance (miles)*	f	Less-than cf
0-9	232	232
10-19	204	436
20-29	63	499
30-39	7	506
40-49	1	507
50-59	1	508
Total	508	

$$Md = L + \left(\frac{\frac{N}{2} - cf}{f} \cdot i \right) = 9.5 + \left(\frac{\frac{508}{2} - 232}{204} \cdot 10 \right)$$

$$= 9.5 + \left(\frac{254 - 232}{204} \cdot 10 \right)$$

$$= 9.5 + \left(\frac{22}{204} \cdot 10 \right) = 9.5 + (.11)(10) = 9.5 + 1.1 = 10.6$$

*Rounded to nearest whole mile.

total of 10 units (19.5 − 9.5). We will then count only a portion of the way across the interval, as indicated by the fraction 22/204. Dividing this fraction to convert it to a decimal, we find that we must count off .11 of the 10 units, or a total of 1.1 (.11 times 10) units. Since the interval begins at its true lower limit of 9.5, counting an additional 1.1 units will place the median at a value of 10.6 miles (9.5 + 1.1).

The formula for the interpolated median presented below provides a convenient summary of this process:

$$Md = L + \left(\frac{\frac{N}{2} - cf}{f} \cdot i \right) \tag{5.1}$$

where Md = median

L = true lower limit of the class interval in which the median is located

N = the total number of observations

cf = cumulated frequency up to but not including the class interval in which the median is located

f = frequency of the class interval in which the median is located

i = width of the class interval in which the median is located

For Table 5.7: $L = 9.5$; $N = 508$; $cf = 232$; $f = 204$; $i = 10$; and the median is calculated as 10.6.

Advantages

The main advantage of the median as a measure of central tendency is that it is an extremely stable measure. That is, unlike the mode, the median is not easily influenced by changes in the way observations are grouped into categories. This is demonstrated by comparing the median for the distribution presented in Table 5.8, in which the six categories from Table 5.7 have been collapsed into three categories, with the median for Table 5.7. The median for Table 5.8 is 11.1, which does not differ greatly from the median value of 10.6 for Table 5.7. Note that $cf = 0$ in Table 5.8 because the median is located in the first class interval.

Another aspect of the stability of the median, which we will be better able to appreciate when we discuss the disadvantages of the mean, is that the median is not easily influenced by the presence of a few extremely low or extremely high values in a distribution. For example, if a 10-year-old patient were added to array A of Table 5.6, the median of the new distribution of 10 patients would decrease only slightly, from 55 to 53. Similarly, if a 90-year-old patient were added to array B of Table 5.6, the median of the new distribution of 9 patients would increase only slightly, from 53 to 55. (These computations may be easily verified by the reader.)

In contrast to the mode, each distribution has one and only one median. Furthermore, since the computation of the

Table 5.8. Obtaining the Median from Grouped Data: Distance to Usual Source of Medical Care, Regrouped

Distance (miles)*	f	Less-than cf
0–19	436	436
20–39	70	506
40–59	2	508
Total	508	

$$Md = L + \left(\frac{\frac{N}{2} - cf}{f} \cdot i\right) = -.5 + \left(\frac{\frac{508}{2} - 0}{436} \cdot 20\right)$$

$$= -.5 + \left(\frac{254 - 0}{436} \cdot 20\right)$$

$$= -.5 + \left(\frac{254}{436} \cdot 20\right) = -.5 + (.58)(20) = -.5 + 11.6 = 11.1$$

*Rounded to nearest whole mile.

median requires ordinal level measurement, the median communicates more information than the mode. This is because the median is located at a very specific, well-defined, reference point within an array or frequency distribution of ordinal or interval level data.

Disadvantages

The main disadvantage of the median is that it becomes uninterpretable when there are many observations that are "tied" for the median rank. This is illustrated in Table 5.9, in which the median age for nine patients is 23. It would be misleading to interpret this value as indicating that half the patients are younger than 23 and the other half are older than 23, for, as we can observe, *none* of the patients are younger than the median age in Table 5.9. This is because all five of the youngest patients have an age equal to that of the median value. Thus there is a five-way tie among these observations for the median rank. In this case the mode would be a more representative, and thus more useful, measure of central tendency than the median, and the mean would be the most useful of all.

In general the fewer the number of categories or values included in a distribution, the greater the likelihood of encountering ties, and the less useful will be the median as a measure of central tendency. Thus, although the median may be calculated with ordinal level data, it is usually most applicable with interval level data, because a large number of ties are frequently encountered with ordinal level variables. For example, classification of patient anxiety levels into only three ordinal categories such as low, medium, and high presents a strong probability that many observations will be tied for the median category, since, if observations were distributed across these categories in a random or equal manner, we would expect approximately one-third of the observations to be tied for the median.

As we have seen, the computation of the median is more

Table 5.9. Array of Patient Ages

23	Median = 23
23	
23	Mode = 23
23	
23	
24	
25	
26	
26	

difficult and time-consuming than that of the mode, particularly in working with grouped data. Also, it is not possible to compute a median for nominal level data. Furthermore, while the stability of the median is its main advantage, the fact that the actual measured value of each observation is not considered in the computation of the median makes it less useful than the mean in many cases. This is especially true when the researcher wishes to include a measure of central tendency in the calculation of further statistical analyses.

Mean

The *mean* is the measure of central tendency with which most people are familiar from everyday usage of the concept of "average," such as average monthly food bill and average miles per gallon of gasoline. In statistics the mean is mathematically defined as the sum of the values of a set of interval level observations divided by the number of observations in the set.

Computation: Ungrouped Data
The mean of a set of ungrouped observations is computed according to the following formula:

$$\bar{X} = \frac{\Sigma X}{N} \tag{5.2}$$

where $\bar{X}$ = mean

ΣX = sum of the observed values

N = total number of observations

Formula 5.2 contains several symbols with which the reader should become very familiar and comfortable, since they are used repeatedly throughout statistics. The symbol $\bar{X}$, which is read as "X bar," is standardly employed to represent the mean of a set of observations. Furthermore, the appearance of the bar symbol (—) above *any* letter is used to indicate the mean of whatever variable is represented by that letter. Thus, if a researcher is studying more than one variable, and the second variable is represented by Y, the symbol $\bar{Y}$ will be used to represent the mean of the observations on the second variable. The capital Greek letter sigma (Σ) is used as a summation sign. Wherever it appears in a formula, it is interpreted as an instruction to sum whatever values follow it. Thus ΣX, which is read as "the sum of X," is an instruction to add up the values of all the observations for variable X. This symbol may also be used to represent the total that is obtained by this summation of

Measures of Central Tendency and Location

23	$\overline{X} = \dfrac{\Sigma X}{N} = \dfrac{216}{9} = 24$
23	
23	
23	
23	
24	
25	
26	
26	

$\Sigma X = 216$
$N = 9$

values. For example, the sum of patient ages presented in
Table 5.10 is 216 years ($\Sigma X = 216$). Finally N, which is already familiar from the computation of the median, is used
to indicate the total number of observations that are included
in a set of data. It is important to recognize that N is equal to
the sum of the frequency column ($N = \Sigma f$) for a set of
grouped data and *not* to the number of categories into which
the observations have been grouped.

The computation of the mean for a set of ungrouped data
is rather straightforward and simple. According to formula
5.2, the mean for the data presented in Table 5.10 is computed as 24.

Computation: Grouped Data

The mean for a set of grouped data is computed according to
the following formula:

$$\overline{X} = \frac{\Sigma fX}{N} \tag{5.3}$$

where $\overline{X}$ = mean

ΣfX = sum of the products of the frequency (f) and
the class midpoint (X) for each class interval

N = total number of observations

While this formula is similar to formula 5.2, two additional
steps are required for the computation of the mean for a set
of grouped data, such as that presented in Table 5.11.

First, since the exact measured value of each observation is
not known, each observation is assigned the value of the mid-

Table 5.11. Obtaining the Mean from Grouped Data: Distance to Usual Source of Medical Care

Distance (miles)*	f	Midpoint (X)	fX
0–9	232	4.5	1044.0
10–19	204	14.5	2958.0
20–29	63	24.5	1543.5
30–39	7	34.5	241.5
40–49	1	44.5	44.5
50–59	1	54.5	54.5
	N = 508		ΣfX = 5886.0

$$\overline{X} = \frac{\Sigma fX}{N} = \frac{5886}{508} = 11.6$$

*Rounded to nearest whole mile.

point of its class interval (X). Second, each class midpoint is multiplied by the frequency of the class interval to take account of the number of observations that have been assigned that value. These values (fX) are then summed and divided by N to obtain the mean. In the case of Table 5.11, the mean has a value of 11.6 miles.

Computation of a Weighted Mean

Situations often arise, especially when working with published data such as the United States Census or Vital and Health Statistics reports, when we are presented with the mean values for each of several subgroups but not for all these groups combined. The combined value can be easily obtained if we are also provided with the number of observations upon which the mean for each subgroup is based. The mean obtained for all the subgroups combined, which is called a *weighted mean*, is computed according to the following formula:

$$\overline{X}_w = \frac{\Sigma n \overline{X}}{N} \tag{5.4}$$

where $\overline{X}_w$ = weighted mean

n = number of observations in each subgroup

$\overline{X}$ = mean of each subgroup

N = total number of observations in all the subgroups combined (Σn)

Table 5.12. Obtaining a Weighted Mean: Mean Number of Physician Visits Made Annually, by Social Class

Subgroup	n	$\overline{X}$	$n\overline{X}$
Lower class	10	3.1	31
Middle class	30	1.5	45
Upper class	15	2.8	42
	$N = 55$		$\Sigma n\overline{X} = 118$

$$\overline{X}_w = \frac{\Sigma n\overline{X}}{N} = \frac{118}{55} = 2.1$$

As illustrated in Table 5.12, the procedure for computing a weighted mean is similar to that for computing a mean for grouped data. The mean for each subgroup is assigned a weight by multiplying it by the number of observations it represents. These values are then summed and divided by the total number of observations to obtain the weighted mean of all groups combined. Thus for Table 5.12 the weighted mean for all three social class groups combined is 2.1 physician visits annually.

It should be noted that, except when the number of observations in each subgroup is equal, it is *incorrect* to obtain the mean for all subgroups combined by simply summing the means for the subgroups and dividing by the number of subgroups. If this were done for Table 5.12, we would obtain the following result for the mean:

$$\frac{3.1 + 1.5 + 2.8}{3} = \frac{7.4}{3} = 2.5$$

The value 2.5 is too high in this case. This is because each of the subgroup means was *wrongly* given an equal weight. Each subgroup does not contribute equally to the total number of observations. Since the middle class subgroup is the largest ($n = 30$), its mean should properly be given the greatest weight in contributing to the combined mean, while the mean of the lower class subgroup, which is the smallest ($n = 10$), should be given the least weight. When the subgroup means are weighted according to their relative contribution to the total number of observations, the mean for all groups combined is pulled down from 2.5 to 2.1 because of the large proportion of observations contributed by the middle class, which has the lowest mean of 1.5 visits.

Advantages
The mean is the most useful measure of central tendency for two reasons. First, it reflects the magnitude or value of every

observation in an interval level data set. That is, each observation contributes to the value of the mean, because the mean is computed by dividing the sum of *all* observations by the total number of observations. By way of contrast it will be recalled that the mode considers only the value of the most frequently occurring observation, while the median considers only the value of the observation that is located in the visual center of a distribution. Thus, the mean takes the fullest advantage of the nature and degree of information available at the interval level of measurement and represents the "typical value" of a distribution. Second, because the mean is derived as the result of arithmetic procedures (i.e., by addition and division rather than by simply counting frequencies and/or ranks as for the mode and median), it can be included in the calculation of further statistical analyses.

While we may sometimes see a distribution that has more than one mode, each distribution will have one and only one mean. Also, unlike the median, for which several observations may be tied, the mean of each distribution will be represented by a unique value.

A convenient aspect of the mean is that it is not necessary to have an entire frequency distribution available in order to compute it. All that is needed are two numbers, the sum of all observations in the distribution (ΣX) and the number of observations in the distribution (N), which are inserted in the formula (5.2) for the calculation of the mean. This is very useful when working with data from a published source such as the United States Census. For example, if we wish to compute the mean number of persons per family in a particular area, we simply consult the census volume for that area, find the total number of persons living in families (ΣX), and divide this figure by the total number of families living in that area.

Disadvantages

While the fact that the mean is sensitive to the value of every observation in a distribution is one of its main advantages, this is also its main disadvantage. To use the mean as a measure of central tendency, we would like it to represent the typical value within a distribution. But the representativeness of the mean in this regard is distorted when a distribution is skewed and includes one or more extreme, or atypical, observations. In such cases the value of the mean is "pulled" in the direction of the extreme observations(s) and will be either lower or higher than it would be if no extreme observations were present. For example, if a 74-year-old patient were added to the array of patient ages presented in Table 5.10, the value of the mean would increase from 24 to 29 ($\Sigma X = 216 + 74 = 290$ and $\overline{X} = 290/10 = 29$). A mean value of 29 would not be a good representative of this array, since only one observation

(74) has a value greater than 26. Thus, the median, which would have a value of 23.5, would be the best representative of the central tendency of this array.

Another disadvantage of the mean is that, since it requires interval level measurement, it cannot be applied to nominal or ordinal level data. As was mentioned in Chapter 2, a large proportion of the variables studied by researchers in nursing and related fields are measured at either the nominal or ordinal level. Therefore the mean cannot be appropriately applied in the analysis of many data sets.

Choosing an Appropriate Measure of Central Tendency

There often arise situations in which it is possible to compute more than one measure of central tendency for a particular data set. A good general rule to follow in deciding which measure of central tendency to use is to select the one that makes the greatest use of the information available. For example, although the only measure of central tendency that may be computed with nominal level data is the mode, both the mode and the median may be computed with ordinal level data. Since the ordinal nature of the data is considered in the computation and is subsequently communicated in the interpretation of the median, the median will be more useful than the mode in most cases. Similarly, although the mode, median, and mean may all be computed for a set of interval level data, the mean will usually be preferred because it considers the value of every observation. The relationship between level of measurement and selection of an appropriate measure of central tendency is summarized in Table 5.13.

Another important point to consider is the nature of the distribution of the data being analyzed. Let us assume that we have measured observations on an interval level variable and therefore can compute all three measures of central tendency that have been discussed in this chapter. Figure 5.1 demonstrates the relative location of these measures for three common types of distribution. When a distribution is symmetrical and unimodal, the mode, median, and mean will all be located at the same point, in the middle of the distribution. For

Table 5.13. Guide to Selection of an Appropriate Measure of Central Tendency According to Level of Measurement

Level of measurement	Measure of central tendency	
	Possible	*Preferred*
Nominal	Mode	Mode
Ordinal	Mode, median	Median
Interval	Mode, median, mean	Mean

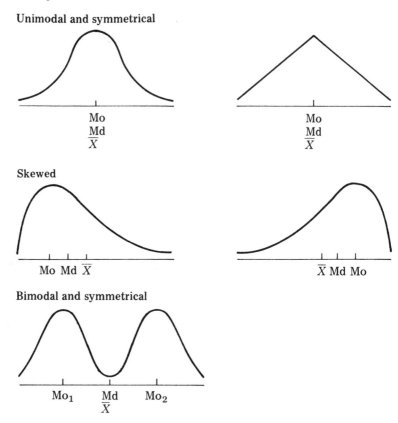

Figure 5.1. Relative location of mode, median, and mean for three common types of distribution.

distributions of this type, the most appropriate measure—the one that will make use of and communicate the greatest amount of available information—is usually selected according to Table 5.13. In a skewed distribution the mode will always be located at the point where the greatest concentration of observations occurs, with the median, and even more the mean, being pulled toward the extreme tail of the distribution. In distributions of this type the selection of the most appropriate measure will often depend upon the purpose to be served in summarizing the distribution. The mode will identify the point where the greatest concentration of observations is located, the median will be located at the visual center and will provide a reference point for dividing the distribution in half, and the mean will indicate the average or central value. Finally, when a distribution is bimodal and symmetrical (or approximately so), both the median and the mean will be located in the middle of the distribution because of its symmetrical nature. In such a case it is very helpful to report the modes, because the median and mean are unable to communicate that a condition of bimodality exists. Furthermore the median and mean may be misleading because few observations are located at or near those values. Of the two, the median may be preferred as a summary descriptive measure because it lets the reader know that half the distribution is below and half is above it.

Of course there is no reason why more than one measure of central tendency may not be reported for a distribution. Although it is contrary to the general goal of summarizing a distribution by presenting a single measure, some distributions may be more adequately described if two or more measures of central tendency are reported for them. For example, reporting the mode and median or mean for a skewed distribution will communicate to the informed reader that the distribution is skewed, because these values will not be equal. Furthermore, if the value of the median or mean is higher than that of the mode, the reader can conclude that the shape of the distribution is a positive skew, while a negative skew is revealed when the median or mean is lower than the mode.

A final note about the use of measures of central tendency: It is not appropriate to compare different measures, because each one communicates a unique type of information about a distribution of observations. Thus it is appropriate only to compare a mode with a mode, a median with a median, and a mean with a mean. Furthermore, unless their distributions are reasonably similar in shape, caution must be exercised even when comparing measures of the same type. For example, Figure 5.2 presents three pairs of oppositely skewed distributions. Without considering the actual shape and location of each distribution, an isolated comparison of the modes of the first pair, the medians of the second pair, and the means of the third pair would lead to the mistaken conclusion that the distributions are approximately, if not exactly, similar for each pair.

Quantiles

In addition to measures of central tendency, *measures of location* are also very useful in providing a summary description of a set of ordinal or interval level data. These measures are so called because they tell us the location of a particular observation relative to that of all the other observations in a distribution. The most commonly used measures of location are collectively referred to as *quantiles*, a name derived from the fact that they divide a given distribution of observations into a specified number of equal parts, or quantities. For example, although we discussed the median as a measure of central tendency in an earlier section of this chapter, the median is also a measure of location and a member of the

Equal modes

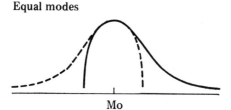

Mo

Equal medians

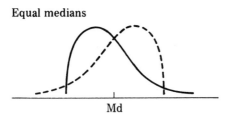

Md

Equal means

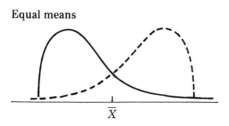

$\overline{X}$

Figure 5.2. Comparison of measures of central tendency for dissimilar distributions.

family of quantiles because it divides a distribution into two equal parts. Although a distribution may be divided into any number of equal parts, in actual practice distributions are most often divided either into fourths or into hundredths, because these divisions have been found to be the most useful. When a distribution is divided into four equal parts, such that one-fourth of the observations are contained in each section, the points or quantiles that separate each fourth are called *quartiles.* The quantiles that divide a distribution into 100 equal parts are called *percentiles.*

It is not appropriate to divide a distribution into quantiles when the number of observations is relatively small, for two reasons. First, only a few observations will be included in each quantile. For example, if a distribution of 20 observations is divided into quartiles, only 5 observations will be included in each. This will tend to obscure any trends that might be present in the data in much the same manner as when a frequency distribution contains an inappropriately large number of categories. Second, the number of quantiles may exceed the number of available observations. Thus, it does not make sense to divide a distribution of less than 100 observations into percentiles, for example. Therefore quantiles are usually computed only when the total number of observations is relatively large. Since it is most convenient to work with a large number of observations in a grouped distribution, this section will discuss the computation of quantiles for grouped data only.

Quartiles

In order to divide a distribution into four equal parts, three points of division must be located. The first quartile (Q_1) is identified as the point that divides a distribution such that one-fourth of the observations are below that point and three-fourths are above it. The second quartile (Q_2) is a point located above the first quartile such that half the observations are below and half are above it. The second quartile should be recognizable from this description as being identical with the median of a distribution. Thus in order to simplify the terminology the second quartile is usually referred to as the *median*. The third quartile (Q_3) is a point located above the median (Q_2) such that three-fourths of the observations are below and one-fourth are above it. The relative location of these measures in a distribution is summarized in Table 5.14. Since the computation of the median was discussed in detail in the previous section, we will be concerned only with the computation of the first and third quartiles here.

The computation of all quantiles follows the same general logic as that which was applied in the calculation of an interpolated median from grouped data, and the similarity between formula 5.1 and those that follow should be apparent. The formula for computing the first quartile is

$$Q_1 = L + \left(\frac{\frac{N}{4} - cf}{f} \cdot i \right)$$
(5.5)

where Q_1 = first quartile

L = true lower limit of the class interval in which the first quartile is located

N = total number of observations

cf = cumulated frequency up to but not including the class interval in which the first quartile is located

f = frequency of the class interval in which the first quartile is located

i = width of the class interval in which the first quartile is located

Table 5.14. Relative Location of Quartiles in a Distribution

Quartile	% Distribution below	% Distribution above
First (Q_1)	25	75
Second (Q_2)/median	50	50
Third (Q_3)	75	25

Two major differences between formula 5.5 and formula 5.1 should be noted. First, they look identical except that in formula 5.5 the expression $N/4$ replaces $N/2$. This is because in order to locate the first quartile we must count only one-fourth of the way into the distribution from the low end. Second, the remaining expressions in formula 5.5 (L, cf, f, and i) refer to the class interval that contains the *first quartile* rather than the median.

The first quartile for Table 5.15 is found by counting

Table 5.15. Obtaining the First and Third Quartiles: Distance to Usual Source of Medical Care

Distance (miles)*	f	Less-than cf
0–9	232	232
10–19	204	436
20–29	63	499
30–39	7	506
40–49	1	507
50–59	1	508
Total	508	

$$Q_1 = L + \left(\frac{\frac{N}{4} - cf}{f} \cdot i \right) = -0.5 + \left(\frac{\frac{508}{4} - 0}{232} \cdot 10 \right)$$

$$= -0.5 + \left(\frac{127 - 0}{232} \cdot 10 \right) = -0.5 + \left(\frac{127}{232} \cdot 10 \right)$$

$$= -0.5 + (.55)(10) = -0.5 + 5.5 = 5$$

$$Q_3 = L + \left(\frac{\frac{3N}{4} - cf}{f} \cdot i \right) = 9.5 + \left(\frac{\frac{1524}{4} - 232}{204} \cdot 10 \right)$$

$$= 9.5 + \left(\frac{381 - 232}{204} \cdot 10 \right) = 9.5 + \left(\frac{149}{204} \cdot 10 \right)$$

$$= 9.5 + (.73)(10) = 9.5 + 7.3 = 16.8$$

*Rounded to nearest whole mile.

$N/4 = 508/4 = 127$ observations into the distribution from the low end. By examining the less-than cumulated frequency column we determine that the first quartile will be located in the 0–9 class interval and that $L = -0.5$, $cf = 0$, $f = 232$, and $i = 10$ accordingly. Inserting these values into formula 5.5 and solving for Q_1, the first quartile is computed as 5 miles. This value is interpreted as indicating that one-fourth, or 25 percent, of the people in the study from which these data are taken reported that they travel *less* than 5 miles to their usual source of medical care and three-fourths, or 75 percent, travel *more* than 5 miles.

The formula for computing the third quartile is

$$Q_3 = L + \left(\frac{\frac{3N}{4} - cf}{f} \cdot i \right) \qquad (5.6)$$

where $Q_3 = $ third quartile

$L = $ true lower limit of the class interval in which the third quartile is located

$N = $ total number of observations

$cf = $ cumulated frequency up to but not including the class interval in which the third quartile is located

$f = $ frequency of the class interval in which the third quartile is located

$i = $ the width of the class interval in which the third quartile is located

This formula is the same as that for computing the first quartile except that in formula 5.6 the expression $N/4$ is replaced by $3N/4$ because the third quartile is located by counting three-fourths of the way into the distribution from the low end. Also, the remaining expressions in formula 5.6 (L, cf, f, and i) refer to the class interval that contains the *third* quartile. For Table 5.15, $L = 9.5$, $3N = 1524$, $cf = 232$, $f = 204$, and $i = 10$. When these values are inserted into formula 5.6, the third quartile is computed as 16.8 miles. This value is interpreted as indicating that three-fourths, or 75 percent, of the respondents travel less than 16.8 miles, and that one-fourth, or 25 percent, travel more than 16.8 miles to their usual source of medical care.

It is important to notice that while the median distance of 10.6 miles (see Table 5.7 for computation) is located between the first and third quartiles, it is not exactly equidistant between them. This is because the median is located by counting off *observations* to the center of a distribution rather than by finding the central value between the lowest and highest values included in a distribution. The median will be located exactly equidistant between the first and third quartiles *only* in the somewhat rare instance when the distribution is unimodal and symmetrical. Also, noting the position of the median between the first and third quartiles will provide a rough idea of the general shape of a distribution without ever examining the distribution directly. As a general rule, if the median is located nearer to the first quartile than it is to the third quartile, this suggests that the distribution is positively skewed; if the median is nearer to the third quartile, this suggests that the distribution is negatively skewed. For Table 5.15 the median is nearer to the first quartile (5.6 miles above) than it is to the third quartile (6.2 miles below), which indicates a concentration of observations in the lower class intervals and suggests that the distribution is positively skewed. This is easily verified by visually inspecting the distribution in Table 5.15.

Quartiles, as are all quantiles, are also useful in comparing two or more distributions the way measures of central tendency are. For example, the distribution in Table 5.15 might be compared with that for another group of subjects in which the first quartile is 3.5 miles and the third quartile is 20 miles. While 25 percent of the respondents in Table 5.15 travel less than 5 miles, the fact that the first quartile for the second distribution is lower suggests that a greater proportion of those in that distribution travel less than 5 miles. On the other hand, since the third quartile for the second distribution is higher than that for Table 5.15, we might conclude that more than 25 percent of the people in the second distribution travel more than 16.8 miles. Thus, while a larger proportion of the members of the second distribution travel a shorter distance than those in Table 5.15, the second distribution also contains a larger proportion of people who travel a longer distance.

Percentiles

To divide a distribution into 100 equal parts, 99 points of division, which are identified as the 1st through the 99th percentiles, must be located. The 1st percentile divides a distribution such that one hundredth, or 1 percent, of the observations are below and 99 hundredths, or 99 percent, are above it, and so on through the 99th percentile, which divides a distribution such that 99 percent of the observations are below and 1 percent are above it. Once again, the median should be recognizable as being identical with the 50th percentile.

The general formula for computing a percentile is

$$P_k = L + \left(\frac{\frac{kN}{100} - cf}{f} \cdot i \right) \tag{5.7}$$

where P_k = kth percentile (k = 1 through 99)

L = true lower limit of the class interval in which the kth percentile is located

N = total number of observations

cf = cumulated frequency up to but not including the class interval in which the kth percentile is located

f = frequency of the class interval in which the kth percentile is located

i = width of the class interval in which the kth percentile is located

For example, the 20th percentile for Table 5.15 is computed as

$$P_{20} = L + \left(\frac{\frac{20N}{100} - cf}{f} \cdot i \right) = -0.5 + \left(\frac{\frac{10,160}{100} - 0}{232} \cdot 10 \right)$$

$$= -0.5 + \left(\frac{101.6 - 0}{232} \cdot 10 \right) = -0.5 + \left(\frac{101.6}{232} \cdot 10 \right)$$

$$= -0.5 + (.44)(10) = -0.5 + 4.4 = 3.9$$

and the 80th percentile is computed as

$$P_{80} = L + \left(\frac{\frac{80N}{100} - cf}{f} \cdot i \right) = 9.5 + \left(\frac{\frac{40,640}{100} - 232}{204} \cdot 10 \right)$$

$$= 9.5 + \left(\frac{406.4 - 232}{204} \cdot 10 \right) = 9.5 + \left(\frac{174.4}{204} \cdot 10 \right)$$

$$= 9.5 + (.85)(10) = 9.5 + 8.5 = 18$$

The 20th percentile indicates that 20 percent of the respondents travel less than 3.9 miles and 80 percent travel more than 3.9 miles, while the 80th percentile indicates that 80 percent travel less than 18 miles and 20 percent travel more than 18 miles.

The uses just described for quartiles are also appropriate to percentiles and therefore will not be repeated. It is worth noting, however, that percentiles are not used just to compare individual observations from two or more distributions but are also often used to compare observations within a single distribution. Perhaps the most common example of this is the reporting of percentile scores on college entrance exams. Percentile scores facilitate comparisons of any individual's performance with that of any or all others who wrote the same exam. Thus a person whose percentile score is 88 performed better than 88 percent of all the others but did not do as well as 12 percent, and a percentile score of 89 is better than a score of 88, and so on. This familiar usage of percentiles leads many persons to regard a high percentile ranking as always good, or desirable, and a low percentile ranking as poor, or undesirable. But this is not true for all variables. In the case of patient stress scores, for example, a *low* percentile ranking is desirable because it indicates a relatively low level of stress, while a high percentile ranking is not desirable. If patients' weights are being considered, then a ranking near the 50th percentile might be most desirable, because a low ranking might indicate that a patient is underweight while a high ranking might indicate overweight.

An alternative to computing quantiles by the use of an interpolation formula is to locate them on a less-than cumulative graph. Although this method yields less precise results than interpolation does, it is usually much quicker and easier (especially if we have already drawn the graph for some other purpose). In Chapter 7 we will discuss yet another method for locating quantiles by the use of the normal distribution table.

WORKING WITH AND INTERPRETING DATA

1. Use the grouped frequency distributions developed for members and nonmembers of La Leche League in question 2, Chapter 3, to compute the following for *each* group:

    a. The mode.
    b. The median (use the interpolation formula).
    c. The mean.

2. Which of the three measures of central tendency you have calculated best represents each group? Briefly justify your answer.

3. Compute the value of the first quartile for each group and compare these values with the first quartile values

that could be obtained by reading from the cumulative frequency graphs constructed for question 2b in Chapter 4.

4. Compute the value of the 90th percentile for each group and compare these values with the 90th percentile values that could be obtained by reading from the cumulative frequency graphs constructed for question 2b in Chapter 4.

5. On the basis of the measures computed in questions 1–4, summarize the comparisons of when members and non-members of La Leche League first introduced solid foods into the diet of their first child.

6. Under what conditions and for what reasons would it be more useful to choose the *mode* rather than the mean as a measure of central tendency for a set of interval level data?

7. Under what conditions and for what reasons would it be more useful to choose the *median* rather than the mean as a measure of central tendency for a set of interval level data?

8. The number and mean birth weight (in pounds) of infants born in each of the four quarters of a year at a community hospital are as follows:

Quarter	n	$\overline{X}$
Jan.–March	10	7.5
April–June	30	6.5
July–Sept.	25	8.0
Oct.–Dec.	15	6.0

Compute the mean birth weight for the total group of 80 infants born in the hospital that year.

9. Triplett, June L. Characteristics and perceptions of low-income women and use of preventive health services: An exploratory study. *Nursing Research* 19:140–146, 1970.

In Table 2 Triplett presents the distribution of good and poor users of preventive health services for several background characteristics. For each characteristic, select the measure of central tendency that would be the most appropriate to describe the distribution of both user groups, and justify your selection.

10. The authors of the following articles report measures of central tendency among their results. Evaluate each

author's use of the measure of central tendency reported. Is the measure appropriate in terms of the level of measurement and the author's purpose? If not, which measure would have been more appropriate and/or useful, and why? Are the results presented in a clear and organized manner?

Chapman, Jacqueline S.   Effects of different nursing approaches upon selected postoperative responses of male herniorrhaphy patients. Pp. 3-14 in Florence S. Downs and Margaret A. Newman (eds.), *A Source Book of Nursing Research*. Philadelphia: Davis, 1973.

Davitz, Lois Jean, and Sidney Harrison Pendleton. Nurses' inferences of suffering. *Nursing Research* 18: 100-107, 1969.

Eoff, Mary Jo Fike, Robert S. Meier, and Carol Miller. Temperature measurement in infants. *Nursing Research* 23:457-460, 1974.

Flaherty, Geraldine G., and Joyce J. Fitzpatrick. Relaxation technique to increase comfort level of postoperative patients. *Nursing Research* 27:352-356, 1978.

Lindeman, Carol A., and Betty Van Aernam.   Nursing intervention with the presurgical patient—the effects of structured and unstructured preoperative teaching. *Nursing Research* 20:319-332, 1971.

Volicer, Beverly, J.   Patients' perceptions of stressful events associated with hospitalization. *Nursing Research* 23:235-238, 1974.

Measures of Variation

The fact that observations vary from one individual to another is what makes a variable interesting. If all observations in a given set were identical, a statistical analysis would be unnecessary, since an examination of any single observation from that data set would reveal what every other observation in the set is like as well. But such uniformity is rarely, if ever, the case in reality. Research consists of an effort to describe, explain, and/or predict variation across a set of observations, and the concept of variation is the foundation of statistical analysis. The techniques discussed in the previous chapters, from simple frequency distributions through tables, graphs, and measures of central tendency and location, are all methods for describing or summarizing how a group of observations vary, or are distributed, across categories or values of a variable.

This chapter discusses several methods for arriving at a single value, generally referred to as a *measure of variation* (variation is also often referred to as *dispersion*), that summarizes the nature and/or degree of variation in a data set. In other words measures of variation indicate how a set of observations are spread out across the various possible categories or values of a variable. Variation is minimum (actually it is nonexistent) when all observations occur in a single category or have the same value. Maximum variation occurs when observations are distributed evenly across all categories or values.

As was the case with the techniques discussed in the previous chapters, the way in which variation is measured depends on the level of measurement of the variable being analyzed. Furthermore each of the measures that will be discussed here is interpretable in reference to one of the measures of central tendency discussed in Chapter 5 and provides a method for evaluating how representative each measure of central tendency is of a particular distribution. The less variation there is, the better any given measure of central tendency represents its distribution. Specifically, the *modal percentage* is interpreted in reference to the mode, the *range* in reference to the median, and *deviation scores* in reference to the mean. Because they are basic conceptual and computational components of many of the most commonly used advanced and inferential statistics, which will be discussed in the following chapters, the major portion of this chapter will be devoted to a discussion of deviation scores about the mean. Finally, a *coefficient of relative variation* will be presented as a convenient method for comparing measures of variation from two or more distributions.

Modal Percentage

An obvious and simple method for evaluating how well the mode represents a distribution is to compute the percentage of observations that are contained in the modal category. When 100 percent of the observations are in the modal category, variation is minimal (in fact, there is *no* variation in this case) and the mode is a perfect summary measure of the distribution. As a rule of thumb, the mode may be considered a good representative of a distribution when at least 50 percent of the observations are in the modal category. The mode is generally not a good representative when the modal category contains less than 50 percent of the observations, because the majority of the observations are not identified with the mode.

Recalling Table 5.1, for example, the modal category, doctor's office, contains 61 percent ($316/515 \times 100$) of the observations and therefore may be considered a fairly good representative of that distribution. In Table 6.1, however, the modal category, 0-9 miles, contains only 46 percent ($232/508 \times 100$) of the observations, indicating that the mode is not a particularly good representative in that case. Furthermore, an almost equally strong concentration of observations (40 percent) is located in the 10-19 category. This supports the decision made in the discussion of Table 5.2 to describe that distribution as bimodal.

The modal percentage is used frequently as a measure of variation for nominal level data, because it is a quick and convenient procedure. A drawback of this method, however, is that while the value of the modal percentage may *theoretically* range from 100 percent to 0 percent, the latter value can *never* be attained in actual practice. This is because by definition the modal category contains the largest frequency or percentage of observations in a distribution. Therefore it is impossible

Table 6.1. Obtaining the Range for an Interval Level Variable: Distance to Usual Source of Care

Distance (miles)*	f
0-9	232
10-19	204
20-29	63
30-39	7
40-49	1
50-59	1
Total	508

Range = −.5 to 59.5 miles, or 60 miles

*Rounded to nearest whole mile.

for the modal category to contain 0 percent of the observations.[1]

Ranges

A range may be computed for ordinal or interval level variables to indicate the location of all or part of a distribution on a measurement scale and/or the number of measurement units that are encompassed by all or part of a distribution. A range is usually interpreted with reference to the median. The most common type of range is the *total range*, which considers an entire distribution. Intermediate ranges of various types are often useful as well. The most frequently used form of intermediate range is the *interquartile range*, which will be discussed in this section.

Total Range

The computation of the total range (usually referred to simply as *the range*) of a distribution involves little more than identifying the true lower limit of the lowest class interval (L) and the true upper limit of the highest class interval (U). For Table 6.1 the true lower limit of the lowest class interval (L) is $-.5$ and the true upper limit of the highest class interval (U) is 59.5. These values may then be used to express the range in either of two ways. First, the range may be reported so as to indicate the location of the distribution on the measurement scale. Thus the distribution presented in Table 6.1 is located between the values $-.5$ and 59.5. Second, the range may be reported as the number of measurement units encompassed by the distribution. This is computed by the simple operation $U - L$, which for Table 6.1 is $59.5 - (-.5) = 60$. This value indicates that the distribution encompasses or is spread across a total of 60 units on the measurement scale.

For ungrouped data, the range is computed by identifying the lowest and highest observations. Thus, for the array of ages of terminally ill patients presented below, the range is located between 40 and 64 and is 24 units ($64 - 40 = 24$) wide.

40
45
48
51
55
56
59
60
64

[1] Although seldom used, probably because its computation is somewhat complex, there is a measure of variation for nominal level variables called the *index of qualitative variation* (IQV), for which values range from

These numbers are not very revealing when considered by themselves. Therefore, when reported for a single distribution, the range is usually reported along with the median, which may be computed for ordinal or interval level data. It is important to note that, while the median is located at the center of a distribution, it is not necessarily located exactly in the center of the range. In fact it rarely is located in the center of the range because the range is not included in the computation of the median. The median for the distribution in Table 6.1 was computed in Chapter 5 as 10.6 miles (see Table 5.7). The location of the median near the low end of the range in this case suggests that the distribution is positively skewed, because half the observations are tightly clustered between the values −.5 and 10.6 while the other half are more widely dispersed between the values 10.6 and 59.5. When the median is located near the high end of the range, it suggests that the distribution is negatively skewed, while a median located near the center of the range suggests a symmetrical distribution.

The range is a convenient measure that is easy to compute. However, it is a relatively crude measure of variation, because it considers only two observations out of an entire distribution and, by itself, tells us nothing about the nature and degree of variation between the two extreme observations. For example, the range for both frequency polygons A (based on Table 6.1) and B in Figure 6.1 is −.5 to 59.5 miles. The distribution of observations within this common range, however, is markedly different for the two data sets.

A major difficulty in dealing with the range is that it is extremely unstable, being subject to variation because of changes in either or both of the extreme low or high observations even though the main part of the distribution remains unchanged. For example, if the observation located in the 50–59 category in Table 6.1 were excluded, the range would be reduced by 10 units from 60 to 50 miles. On the other hand, the size of the range would be doubled if a single observation with a value of 120 miles were added to Table 6.1. In this last example the total range presents the impression that a much greater degree of variation exists among the observations than is actually the case. Therefore, when presented with a data set for which the range appears to be large, it may be useful to examine the frequency distribution of the data directly (by constructing a frequency polygon for example) to determine whether the size of the range is inflated by the presence of a few extremely high or low observations.

---

0 to +1.00. The IQV is computed as the ratio of observed variation to the maximum possible variation for a given distribution and is discussed in detail in Mueller, Schuessler, and Costner (1977).

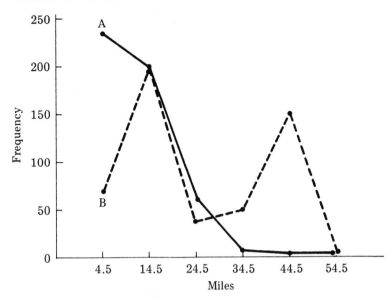

For both A and B: $n = 508$
Range $= -0.5$ to 59.5

Figure 6.1. Comparison of two distributions with equal range and equal n.

Interquartile Range

An effective method for compensating for the instability of the total range is to compute one of several intermediate ranges, which exclude an equal portion of the observations at each end of a distribution and include only the more typical and reliable observations located toward the center.[2] The most commonly employed intermediate range is the interquartile range, which is computed by identifying the first and third quartiles and finding the range between them. Thus the interquartile range encompasses the middle 50 percent of a distribution.

In the discussion of Table 5.15 the first and third quartiles were computed for the data presented in Table 6.1 as 5 and 16.8 miles respectively. Thus the interquartile range for Table 6.1 is located between these values and encompasses 11.8 units on the measurement scale. Although the earlier analysis of the median and total range indicated a positively skewed distribution, the median of 10.6 is located almost midway within the interquartile range. This indicates that the distribution is only slightly skewed by the presence of a few extremely

---

[2] The reliability of the extreme observations is sometimes questioned by researchers because, although they may be entirely valid and accurate, there is a strong possibility that such atypical observations are the result of measurement error or represent rare events that should be analyzed separately.

Table 6.2. Summing Deviation Scores about the Mean: Age of Terminally Ill Patients

X	$X - \overline{X}$	
40	−11.75	
45	−6.75	
48	−3.75	−23
51	−0.75	
55	3.25	
56	4.25	
59	7.25	+23
60	8.25	
$\Sigma X = 414$	$\Sigma(X - \overline{X}) = 0.00$	

$$\overline{X} = \frac{\Sigma X}{N} = \frac{414}{8} = 51.75$$

high observations, while a major portion of the distribution is symmetrically distributed about the median within a relatively narrow range of values. In general the more narrow the interquartile range, the more peaked a distribution is, because half the observations are condensed across fewer units on the measurement scale.

Deviation Scores About the Mean

When the mean has been selected as the measure of central tendency for a distribution of interval level data, several alternatives are available for summarizing how the observations vary with reference to the mean value. A major advantage of interval level data is that the exact number of measurement units that separate *each* observation from the mean may be specified arithmetically by subtracting the mean from the value of each observation. This procedure $(X - \overline{X})$ yields a *deviation score* that is positive for observations larger than the mean and negative for those smaller than the mean.[3] A unique characteristic of the mean is that, for any distribution, the sum of the arithmetic deviations from it is always equal to zero.[4] As demonstrated in Table 6.2, some deviation scores are positive and others are negative. The mean, which was described in the previous chapter as the central value of a

[3] The value $X - \overline{X}$ is often symbolized as x.
[4] This sum will occasionally not be exactly equal to zero, although it will be very close to zero. Such slight variations are the result of rounding error and can be tolerated with no serious effect upon the results of the analysis.

distribution, is located such that the sum of the positive scores equals that of the negative scores. The net result of this balance among deviation scores is that they sum to zero. Thus the sum of the arithmetic deviations about the mean is useless as a measure of variation, because it cannot distinguish between distributions in which the pattern and degree of variation are different.

Average Deviation

A simple method for computing a measure of variation based upon deviations about the mean is to sum the absolute values of the deviation scores, ignoring positive and negative signs. When this sum, which will always be positive, is divided by the total number of observations, as in the formula 6.1, the *average deviation* is obtained.

$$\text{AD} = \frac{\Sigma |X - \overline{X}|}{N} \tag{6.1}$$

where AD = average deviation

$|X - \overline{X}|$ = absolute value of the deviation score for each observation

N = total number of observations

This value is interpretable as the average number of measurement units separating any observation and the mean. Thus the average number of units separating any observation and the mean for Table 6.3 is 5.75 years.

The average deviation has a great deal of intuitive meaning as a measure of variation that takes into account the value of every observation in a distribution of interval data. However, because absolute values are not easily manipulated arithmetically, the average deviation is rarely used in further statistical analyses.

Sum of Squares

The most common method for simultaneously avoiding the zero-sum problem encountered with arithmetic deviations in order to perform further computations is to square each deviation score. The square of either a positive or a negative number is always positive. Therefore the sum of the squared deviations about the mean, commonly called the *sum of squares*, will always be positive and greater than zero. According to formula 6.2, the sum of squares (SS) for Table 6.4 is 347.48.

$$\text{SS} = \Sigma (X - \overline{X})^2 \tag{6.2}$$

Table 6.3. Obtaining Average Deviation: Age of Terminally Ill Patients

X	$|X - \overline{X}|$
40	11.75
45	6.75
48	3.75
51	0.75
55	3.25
56	4.25
59	7.25
60	8.25
$\Sigma X = 414$	$\Sigma|X - \overline{X}| = 46.00$

$$\overline{X} = \frac{\Sigma X}{N} = \frac{414}{8} = 51.75$$

$$AD = \frac{\Sigma|X - \overline{X}|}{N} = \frac{46}{8} = 5.75$$

Table 6.4. Obtaining Sum of Squares, Variance, and Standard Deviation for Ungrouped Data: Age of Terminally Ill Patients

X	$X - \overline{X}$	$(X - \overline{X})^2$
40	−11.75	138.06
45	−6.75	45.56
48	−3.75	14.06
51	−0.75	0.56
55	3.25	10.56
56	4.25	18.06
59	7.25	52.56
60	8.25	68.06
$\Sigma X = 414$		$\Sigma(X - \overline{X})^2 = 347.48$

$$\overline{X} = \frac{\Sigma X}{N} = \frac{414}{8} = 51.75$$

$$SS = \Sigma(X - \overline{X})^2 = 347.48$$

$$\sigma^2 = \frac{\Sigma(X - \overline{X})^2}{N} = \frac{347.48}{8} = 43.44$$

$$\sigma = \sqrt{\frac{\Sigma(X - \overline{X})^2}{N}} = \sqrt{\frac{347.48}{8}} = \sqrt{43.44} = 6.59$$

The value of the sum of squares may range from zero to infinity. The larger the value, the more variation is present in a data set. A sum of squares value is not very meaningful by itself and is almost always interpreted by means of comparison with the sums of squares for other distributions of interest to the researcher.

Although the sum of squares does not have an immediate and strong intuitive appeal, it is an extremely valuable and important measure that will be encountered frequently in subsequent chapters. The main feature of the sum of squares, and the characteristic that makes it extremely useful in further analyses, is that the value of the sum of the squared deviations about the mean is smaller than the value of the sum of the squared deviations that might be computed about any other value selected from a given distribution. This rule that the sum of squares about the mean is minimal is called the *least-squares principle*. The importance and application of this rule will become apparent especially in the discussion of linear regression in Chapter 13.

Variance

Another measure of variation about the mean that is useful in further analyses is the *variance*. As indicated in formula 6.3, the variance (σ^2) is computed by dividing the sum of squares by the total number of observations in a distribution.[5]

$$\sigma^2 = \frac{\Sigma(X - \overline{X})^2}{N} \tag{6.3}$$

Thus the variance is interpretable as the *average sum of squares*. For Table 6.4, the variance is computed as 43.44. The value of the variance may range from zero to infinity and, like the sum of squares, the variance for different distributions may be compared to determine where variance is the greatest.

Standard Deviation

When deviation scores are squared in the computation of the sum of squares and variance, the measurement scale is shifted from the original linear scale to a geometric scale. A return to the linear scale may be achieved by performing the mathematical operation that is the opposite of squaring, that is, finding the square root. Thus, according to formula 6.4, the standard deviation (σ) is computed as the square root of the variance and has a value of 6.59 in Table 6.4.[6]

$$\sigma = \sqrt{\frac{\Sigma(X - \overline{X})^2}{N}} \tag{6.4}$$

---

[5] The symbol σ is the lowercase form of the Greek letter sigma (Σ).
[6] Although a square root may be either positive or negative, the standard deviation is always reported as a positive value.

Computational Shortcuts

There is an alternative to the rather lengthy procedure of finding each deviation score and squaring it before computing the sum of squares, variance, or standard deviation. Computational formulas, which are derived from formulas 6.2, 6.3, and 6.4, are available that simplify the computation of these measures (especially when the computations are performed on a calculator).[7] These were not introduced initially in this discussion, however, because they obscure the concept underlying the use of squared deviations to measure variation about the mean.

The computation of the sum of squares is simplified when performed according to formula 6.5.

$$SS = \Sigma X^2 - \frac{(\Sigma X)^2}{N} \tag{6.5}$$

As illustrated in Table 6.5, this formula yields virtually the same value, 347.5, as that obtained in Table 6.4 (347.48) for the same set of data. The very slight difference is attributable to rounding error.

The variance is conveniently computed according to formula 6.6, which yields exactly the same result of 43.44 for Table 6.5 as was obtained for Table 6.4.

$$\sigma^2 = \frac{\Sigma X^2}{N} - \overline{X}^2 \tag{6.6}$$

Similarly, according to formula 6.7, the standard deviation is computed as 6.59 for Table 6.5, which is identical with the result previously obtained for Table 6.4.

$$\sigma = \sqrt{\frac{\Sigma X^2}{N} - \overline{X}^2} \tag{6.7}$$

Computation: Grouped Data

As for the computation of a mean for grouped data (see Chapter 5), the computation of the sum of squares, variance, and standard deviation for a set of grouped data requires that the squared deviations be multiplied by the frequency of their corresponding class interval. Thus the conceptual formulas for these measures are as follows:

$$SS = \Sigma f(X - \overline{X})^2 \tag{6.8}$$

$$\sigma^2 = \frac{\Sigma f(X - \overline{X})^2}{N} \tag{6.9}$$

$$\sigma = \sqrt{\frac{\Sigma f(X - \overline{X})^2}{N}} \tag{6.10}$$

[7] The derivations are not presented here. Interested readers should see Blalock (1972).

Table 6.5. Computational Shortcut for Obtaining Sum of Squares, Variance, and Standard Deviation for Ungrouped Data: Age of Terminally Ill Patients

X	X^2
40	1,600
45	2,025
48	2,304
51	2,601
55	3,025
56	3,136
59	3,481
60	3,600
$\Sigma X = 414$	$\Sigma X^2 = 21,772$

$$\overline{X} = \frac{\Sigma X}{N} = \frac{414}{8} = 51.75$$

$$SS = \Sigma X^2 - \frac{(\Sigma X)^2}{N} = 21,772 - \frac{414^2}{8} = 21,772 - \frac{171,396}{8}$$

$$= 21,772 - 21,424.5 = 347.5$$

$$\sigma^2 = \frac{\Sigma X^2}{N} - \overline{X}^2 = \frac{21,772}{8} - 51.75^2 = 2721.5 - 2678.06 = 43.44$$

$$\sigma = \sqrt{\frac{\Sigma X^2}{N} - \overline{X}^2} = \sqrt{\frac{21,772}{8} - 51.75^2} = \sqrt{2721.5 - 2678.06}$$

$$= \sqrt{43.44} = 6.59$$

The following computational formulas are more commonly used, however, because they simplify the computational process considerably:

$$SS = \Sigma f X^2 - \frac{(\Sigma f X)^2}{N} \tag{6.11}$$

$$\sigma^2 = \frac{\Sigma f X^2}{N} - \overline{X}^2 \tag{6.12}$$

$$\sigma = \sqrt{\frac{\Sigma f X^2}{N} - \overline{X}^2} \tag{6.13}$$

Accordingly, for Table 6.6 the sum of squares is computed as 30,488.19, the variance as 59.71, and the standard deviation as 7.73. The reader may wish to verify that, according to the conceptual formulas (formulas 6.8, 6.9, and 6.10), the sum of squares for Table 6.6 is computed as 30,488.28, the variance

Table 6.6 Obtaining Sum of Squares, Variance, and Standard Deviation for Grouped Data: Distance to Usual Source of Care

Distance (miles)*	f	(Midpoint) X	fX	X^2	fX^2
0-9	232	4.5	1044.0	20.25	4,698.00
10-19	204	14.5	2958.0	210.25	42,891.00
20-29	63	24.5	1543.5	600.25	37,815.75
30-39	7	34.5	241.5	1190.25	8,331.75
40-49	1	44.5	44.5	1980.25	1,980.25
50-59	1	54.5	54.5	2970.25	2,970.25
	$N = 508$		$\Sigma fX = 5886.0$		$\Sigma fX^2 = 98,687.00$

$$\overline{X} = \frac{\Sigma fX}{N} = \frac{5886}{508} = 11.6$$

$$SS = \Sigma fX^2 - \frac{(\Sigma fX)^2}{N} = 98,687 - \frac{5,886^2}{508} = 98,687 - 68,198.81 = 30,488.19$$

$$\sigma^2 = \frac{\Sigma fX^2}{N} - \overline{X}^2 = \frac{98,687}{508} - 11.6^2 = 194.27 - 134.56 = 59.71$$

$$\sigma = \sqrt{\frac{\Sigma fX^2}{N} - \overline{X}^2} = \sqrt{\frac{98,687}{508} - 11.6^2} = \sqrt{194.27 - 134.56} = \sqrt{59.71} = 7.73$$

*Rounded to nearest whole mile.

as 60.02, and the standard deviation as 7.75. Again, both sets of formulas yield very similar results, the slight differences being attributable to rounding error.

Interpretation of the Standard Deviation
Of all measures of variation discussed in this chapter the standard deviation may be considered to be the most important, because it is used in advanced statistical computations more often than the others. Unfortunately a nagging problem regarding the standard deviation is that it has no clear intuitive meaning. This abstract characteristic understandably leaves many students with an uneasy feeling regarding the standard deviation. However, the utility and interpretation of the standard deviation will be better appreciated when standard scores and the normal distribution are discussed in the next chapter.

For the present the standard deviation may be understood simply as a unit of measure of the variation among a set of interval observations. Thus, given two distributions with similar means, the distribution with the larger standard deviation has the greater degree of variation, indicating that its mean is not as good a representative of central tendency as the mean of the distribution with the smaller standard deviation. For example, one might compare the distribution in Table 6.6, which has a mean of 11.6 and a standard deviation of 7.73, with the distribution of distance to usual source of care for another group of subjects. Suppose that for this second distribution the mean is 12.5 and the standard deviation is

4.29. Because the mean for the second distribution is slightly higher than that for Table 6.6, this indicates that *overall* the subjects in the second distribution travel slightly longer distances. But the fact that the standard deviation is smaller for this group indicates that more of its members travel a distance equal or near to the mean than is the case for Table 6.6. Thus, while some members of the second group travel a longer distance, others travel a shorter distance to their usual source of care than the members of the first group.

The standard deviation will usually equal approximately one-sixth the size of the range for most distributions. This is roughly true for Table 6.6, where one-sixth of the range of 60 miles is equal to 10 and the standard deviation is almost 8 miles (7.73). This relationship is useful because it provides a rough but convenient method for estimating the expected value of the standard deviation and thus for checking the accuracy of the computed value.

Another useful rule of thumb is that for *any* distribution, regardless of its shape, at least 75 percent of the observations will fall within two standard deviations below and above the mean.[8] For Table 6.6, two times the standard deviation equals 15.46. Subtracting and adding this value from and to the mean reveals that at least 75 percent of the distribution can be expected to fall between 0 (actually −3.86) and 27.06 miles. This is verified by noting that more than 86 percent (232 + 204 ÷ 508) of this distribution falls within this range.

Finally, the value of the standard deviation varies from distribution to distribution. Although two distributions may have the same mean, they do not necessarily also have the same standard deviation. In fact this will rarely be the case. For example, the distribution in Table 6.7 has exactly the same mean as that in Table 6.5 (51.75) but has a larger standard deviation (10.00 as compared with 6.59).

Comparing Measures of Variation

Just as different measures of central tendency may not be compared with each other, neither can comparisons be made between different measures of variation from two or more distributions. This of course is because each measure is conceived and computed in a unique way and therefore communicates a unique kind of information regarding the variation among a set of observations.

Also one must be careful about comparing measures of variation for two distributions when the number of observations contained in each is not similar. This is because variation is unstable in distributions that contain a small number of

[8] This is called Chebyshev's theorem and is discussed in detail in Loether and McTavish, p. 149 (1974).

Table 6.7. Obtaining Standard Deviation for Age of Terminally Ill Patients

X	X^2
38	1,444
39	1,521
43	1,849
50	2,500
57	3,249
61	3,721
62	3,844
64	4,096
$\Sigma X = 414$	$\Sigma X^2 = 22,224$

$$\bar{X} = \frac{\Sigma X}{N} = \frac{414}{8} = 51.75$$

$$\sigma = \sqrt{\frac{\Sigma X^2}{N} - \bar{X}^2} = \sqrt{\frac{22,224}{8} - 51.75^2} = \sqrt{2778 - 2678.06}$$

$$= \sqrt{99.94} = 10.00$$

observations, since each observation accounts for a relatively large proportion of the total variation. For example, in a distribution of 20 observations each observation represents 5 percent of the entire distribution. Thus a change in the value of a single observation will be reflected by a change in 5 percent of the distribution and a change in only two observations will be reflected by a change in 10 percent of the distribution. In such cases, a measure of variation can be greatly influenced by the presence of only one or two atypical observations. Therefore variation should be compared across distributions only when they contain approximately equal numbers of observations, so that the stability or reliability of measures of their variation is similar. Furthermore, because variation is highly unstable when the number of observations is very small, less than 10 for example, it may be misleading to attempt any comparison of measures of variation at all.

Another consideration is that even when two distributions contain similar and relatively large numbers of observations, both distributions should occupy similar positions along the measurement scale. Consider, for example, two distributions of patients' weights. One distribution contains the weights of 100 infants and has a mean of 7 pounds and a standard deviation of 2 pounds. The other distribution contains the weights of 100 adults and has a mean of 150 pounds and a standard deviation of 30 pounds. Although most people would recognize the general absurdity of comparing the means for these distributions, the fact that a direct comparison of their standard deviations is equally useless is not so apparent. Many observers would be quick to conclude that, since the standard deviation is much smaller for the infants, there is less variation within that distribution and the mean is more representative than among the adult distribution. This conclusion would be fallacious, however, because, as a general rule, the larger the value of the mean, the larger the value of the standard deviation. That is, the value of the mean and standard deviation of the adult distribution is large by virtue of the position on the measurement scale where adult weight is located.

The influence of scale location may be taken into account by the *coefficient of relative variation* (CRV), which is computed as the ratio between a measure of variation and its associated measure of central tendency. Thus the coefficient of relative variation for the standard deviation is computed by dividing it by the mean. The CRV for the distribution of the infants' weights is .29 (2 ÷ 7) and is .20 (30 ÷ 150) for the distribution of the adults' weights. This reveals that, relative to their positions on the measurement scale, the distribution of the infants' weights displays more variation than that of the adults' weights.

A coefficient of relative variation may be computed for other measures of variation as well. For example, the CRV for the average deviation, sum of squares, and variance is computed by dividing by the mean, because these are measures of variation about the mean of a distribution. A CRV may be similarly computed for the total range and the interquartile range by dividing by the median. It is not possible to compute a CRV for nominal level distributions, because the concept of scale location does not apply. Because there are so many different ways to compute a coefficient of relative variation, it is important to specify how the coefficient was computed whenever it is reported.

WORKING WITH AND INTERPRETING DATA

1. Continue your analysis of when members and nonmembers of La Leche League first introduced solid foods into the diet of their first child, and compute the following measures of variation for both members and nonmembers:

   a. Modal percentage.
   b. Total range in terms of both location and size.
   c. Interquartile range in terms of both location and size.
   d. Standard deviation.

2. How does the additional information from question 1 above add to your summary and comparison of these groups as stated in answer to question 5 in Chapter 5?

3. Returning to your answer to question 2 in Chapter 5, how do these measures of variation assist you in selecting the most appropriate measure of central tendency?

4. Which group, members or nonmembers, displays the greatest degree of variation according to your computations in question 1?

5. For each of the following data sets indicate whether the general shape of the distribution is symmetrical, a positive skew, or a negative skew, and briefly justify your answer.

   a. Survival time (in months) for 50 patients who received a new treatment for lung cancer:
      Mode = 10   Modal percentage = 45%
      Median = 14   Total range = 2-51
      Mean = 17   Standard deviation = 85

   b. Percent recommended daily allowance (RDA) caloric intake for 60 elderly patients:
      Mode = 75   Modal percentage = 55%
      Median = 70   Total range = 20-90
      Mean = 55   Standard deviation = 7

   c. Weight (in pounds) of 25 female patients:
      Mode = 130   Modal percentage = 68%
      Median = 130   Total range = 90-170
      Mean = 130   Standard deviation = 7

   d. Length of hospital stay (in days) for 32 surgical patients:
      Mode = 7   Modal percentage = 21%
      Median = 5   Total range = 2-11
      Mean = 4.2   Standard deviation = 3.5

6. If two distributions have the same total range and mean, would you conclude that the distributions are identical? Justify your answer.

7. Refer again to the article by Triplett (see question 9 in Chapter 5) and select the appropriate measure of variation for each background characteristic displayed in Table 2 of that article. Remember to take the measure of central tendency you selected in question 9, Chapter 5, into consideration. Justify your choice.

8. The authors of the following articles report measures of variation among their results. Evaluate each author's use of the measure of variation reported. Is the measure appro-

priate considering the measure of central tendency reported? If not, which measure would have been more appropriate, and why?

Chapman, Jacqueline S.   Effects of different nursing approaches upon selected postoperative responses of male herniorrhaphy patients. Pp. 3–14 in Florence S. Downs and Margaret A. Newman (eds.), *A Source Book of Nursing Research*. Philadelphia: Davis, 1973.
Davitz, Lois Jean, and Sidney Harrison Pendleton. Nurses' inferences of suffering. *Nursing Research* 18:100–107, 1969.

Especially note Table 4 in this article. On the basis of a comparison of the means and standard deviations presented, which clinical specialty differs the most from the others?

Eoff, Mary Jo Fike, Robert S. Meier, and Carol Miller. Temperature measurement in infants. *Nursing Research* 23:457–460, 1974.

From the results presented in Table 2 of this article, which instrument/method combination produces the most consistent measurements?

Gerber, Rose Marie, and Suzanne Rowe Van Ort. Topical application of insulin in decubitus ulcers. *Nursing Research* 28:16–19, 1979.

Compare the experimental and control group data presented in Table 2 of this article. Does your interpretation agree with that of the authors?

Standard Scores and the Normal Distribution

Two important and related concepts, standard scores and the normal distribution, are introduced in this chapter. An understanding of these concepts will allow us to elaborate upon the application and interpretation of the standard deviation and will provide a basis for the introduction to inferential statistics that is presented in Chapter 8. After each concept is introduced separately, this chapter will present several basic approaches to how standard scores and the normal distribution may be applied in combination with each other in statistical analyses.

Standard Scores

The most common and important application of the standard deviation is in the computation of standard scores (often referred to as z scores). Standard scores are a method for transforming or expressing interval level observations in terms of standard deviation units. This is accomplished by computing the arithmetic deviation (maintaining the plus or minus sign) of the observation from the mean of its distribution and then dividing the deviation score by the standard deviation. When computed according to formula 7.1

$$z = \frac{X - \overline{X}}{\sigma} \tag{7.1}$$

a z score of 0 indicates that an observation is equal to the mean because the z score will equal 0 when $X - \overline{X} = 0$. When $X - \overline{X} = \sigma$, the z score will equal $+1.00$, indicating that the observation is one standard deviation *above* the mean. When $X - \overline{X} = 2\sigma$, the z score will equal $+2.00$, indicating that the observation is two standard deviations above the mean, and so on. Similarly, for negative values, when $X - \overline{X} = -\sigma$, the z score will equal -1.00, indicating that the observation is one standard deviation *below* the mean. When $X - \overline{X} = -1.5\sigma$, the z score will equal -1.50, indicating that the observation is one and one-half standard deviations below the mean, and so on. Thus the z score is a very effective method of comparing observations from either the same or different distributions, because it accounts for both the amount and direction of variation of each observation from the mean in a standardized manner by using standard deviation units as a common basis of comparison.

For example, recall the distribution of adults' weights discussed in the previous chapter, in which the mean is 150 pounds with a standard deviation equal to 30. According to formula 7.1, the z score for a person weighing 125 pounds is -0.83 ($125 - 150 \div 30$) and the z score for a person weighing 185 pounds is $+1.17$ ($185 - 150 \div 30$). If we ignore the fact that we know the value of the mean for this distribution and consider only these z score values, we can draw two important conclusions. First, the signs of the z scores indicate that the person who weighs 125 pounds is below the mean (negative sign) and the person who weighs 185 pounds is above the mean (positive sign). Second, the magnitude of the values indicates that the person weighing 185 pounds is farther away from the mean (1.17 standard deviation units) than the person weighing 125 pounds (.83 standard deviation units) and thus is less typical of the distribution.

Furthermore, z scores enable us to make comparisons between observations from the adult weight distribution and observations from the distribution of weight for a group of infants, for which the mean is 7 with a standard deviation of 2. The z score for an infant weighing 12.6 pounds is $+2.80$ ($12.6 - 7 \div 2$), indicating that it is 2.80 standard deviation units above the mean. Since the magnitude of this z score is larger than that for the 185-pound adult ($z = +1.17$), it can be concluded that the 12.6-pound infant is "heavier" *relative to its distribution* than the 185-pound adult.

Both standard scores and the standard deviation have a wider application and interpretation when they are used with the normal distribution. Therefore we will return to the topic of standard scores following an introduction to the normal distribution.

The Normal Distribution

The normal distribution is a very important concept, because it is the basis for probability sampling theory (so-called random sampling) and inferential statistics, whereby a researcher attempts to generalize from results observed in a sample to the population represented by that sample. Although probability sampling is not formally discussed at length in this book, a brief introduction to sampling theory is provided in the next chapter. Before discussing the properties of the normal distribution it is important to note that the word "normal" in the name of this distribution is no more than part of a name. It should not be taken to imply that other types of distributions are to be regarded as unusual or defective in any manner. In fact most distributions encountered in actual practice are *not* "normal distributions." Actually it is impossible to observe a *true* normal distribution, because the normal distribution in its purest form is a theoretical mathematical model.

Graphically the normal distribution is described by the so-called bell-shaped curve depicted in Figure 7.1. Some

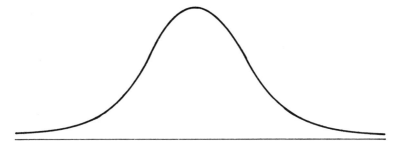

Figure 7.1. Shape of the normal distribution.

readers may be familiar with it from having taken a course in which the instructor determined the final grade distribution "on a curve." Visual inspection of Figure 7.1 reveals four basic properties of the normal distribution. First, the normal distribution contains an infinite number of observations ($N = \infty$) as indicated by the fact that the curve will never intersect with the baseline or horizontal axis. Second, it is unimodal, that is, it has only one distinct mode. Third, it is perfectly symmetrical, meaning that if the curve were divided at the median, two identical but reversed halves would be obtained. From these last two properties it follows that all three measures of central tendency discussed in Chapter 5, the mode, median, and mean, are identical and are located at the exact center of the normal distribution. Fourth, most of the values are close to the mean, with values that are relatively small or large in relation to the mean occurring infrequently.

For the sake of convenience in computations mathematicians have assigned the mean (and thus also the mode and median) of the normal distribution the value of zero. The value of the standard deviation of the normal distribution has been defined as equal to 1.00. The rationale for assigning the values 0 and 1.00 to the mean and standard deviation respectively is to facilitate the use of standard scores (z scores) in reference to the normal distribution. The conversion of the mean of the normal distribution (which equals zero) to a z score yields the result

$$z = \frac{X - \overline{X}}{\sigma} = \frac{0 - 0}{1.00} = \frac{0}{1.00} = 0$$

and the conversion of the standard deviation of the normal distribution (which equals 1.00) to a z score yields

$$z = \frac{X - \overline{X}}{\sigma} = \frac{1.00 - 0}{1.00} = \frac{1.00}{1.00} = 1.00$$

Thus there is a perfect correspondence between actual values on the normal distribution and their z scores. This conveniently

combines two types of information into a single value. The
reader can similarly verify that this relationship applies to
any value for the normal distribution. For example, the value
-2.37 can also be directly interpreted as a z score indicating
that the value is 2.37 standard deviation units below the
mean of zero for the normal distribution, while the value
$+1.96$ is 1.96 standard deviation units above the mean. For
this reason it is standard practice to identify points or values
along the normal distribution in terms of z scores, as illustrated in Figure 7.2.

What makes the normal distribution so useful in statistics
is the fact that mathematicians have computed the percentage of the normal distribution that is located at virtually any
point along the normal curve. For example, as depicted in
Figure 7.3, it is known that 34.13 percent of the normal
distribution is located between the mean and one standard
deviation either below ($z = -1.00$) or above ($z = +1.00$) it.
By adding these two percentages together we find that 68.26
percent of the normal distribution is located between the
points which are one standard deviation unit below and
above the mean as illustrated in Figure 7.4. Figure 7.3 also
indicates that 13.59 percent of the normal distribution is
located between the points that are one and two standard
deviation units either below or above the mean. By addition

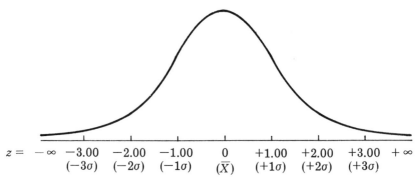

Figure 7.2. Major points along the normal distribution.

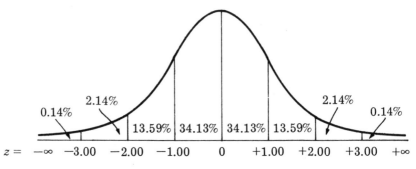

Figure 7.3. Percentage of the normal distribution between major
points.

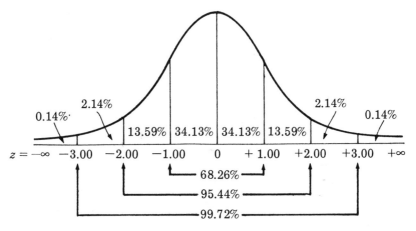

Figure 7.4. Percentage of the normal distribution between −1.00 and +1.00, −2.00 and +2.00, and −3.00 and +3.00.

we can determine that 47.72 percent (34.13 + 13.59) of the normal distribution is located between the mean and a point that is two standard deviation units either below or above it, as illustrated in Figure 7.5. Also, as shown in Figure 7.4, 95.44 percent (47.72 + 47.72) is located between the points that are two standard deviation units below and above the mean. Continuing our examination of Figure 7.3 we can also observe that 2.14 percent of the normal distribution is located between the points that are two and three standard deviation units below or above the mean, and by addition that 49.86 percent (34.13 + 13.59 + 2.14) is between the mean and a point three standard deviation units below or above it (see Figure 7.5). This leaves only 0.14 percent (50.00% − 49.86%) of the normal distribution that is located more than three standard deviation units below or above the mean. It is also important to note in Figure 7.4 that 99.72 percent (49.86% + 49.86%) of the normal distribution is located between the points that are three standard deviation

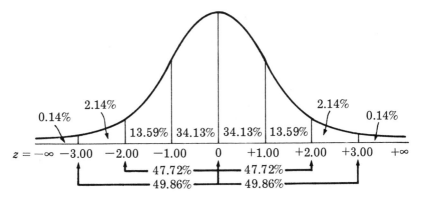

Figure 7.5. Percentage of the normal distribution between the mean and major points.

units below and above the mean. Therefore, although points along the normal distribution range from minus infinity $(-\infty)$ to plus infinity $(+\infty)$, there are not many occasions when we are concerned with z scores with a value greater than ± 3.00, because almost all the normal distribution is located between these points.

In addition to 0, ± 1.00, ± 2.00, and ± 3.00 there are many other points along the normal distribution curve. In fact the number is infinite. It is standard practice, however, to round a computed z score value to the nearest hundredth, because little advantage is gained from carrying the computation out to more than two places to the right of the decimal point.

Normal Distribution Table

The normal distribution is particularly easy to use because mathematicians have compiled tables that display the proportion of the normal distribution that is located at various points along the curve. Table C.2 (in Appendix C of this book) displays the proportion of the normal distribution that is located below or above a given z score value depending on whether the sign of the z score is negative or positive, respectively. Another way of describing Table C.2 is that it displays the proportion of the normal distribution that is located in either the negative or the positive tail of the normal curve that is determined by a particular z score. As will be seen in the following chapters, Table C.2 is a basic tool in inferential statistics and the process of hypothesis testing.

The format of this table is different from the cross-classification tables discussed in Chapter 3, and some explanation regarding how to read it is necessary. Table C.2 contains two kinds of numbers, z scores and proportions. The proportions are presented in the center or body of the table, while the z scores are listed in the left and top margins. In order to save space, the z score values have been split apart in the table, with the first two digits being listed in the left margin and the third digit listed in the top margin. Also, no distinction is made between negative and positive z scores, because the proportions in the body of the table apply equally to both the negative and the positive halves of the curve, since the normal distribution is perfectly symmetrical.

For example, to find the proportion of the normal distribution that is located beyond a z score of $+1.96$, find the first two digits, 1.9, in the left margin and mark this location with the index finger of your left hand. Next, find the third digit of the z score, which is 6, in the top margin, and mark its location with the index finger of your right hand. Now move your left index finger along the row corresponding to 1.9 in the left margin until you come to the column labeled 6 in the top margin. At this point you should read the number .0250, which is the proportion of the normal distribution that is

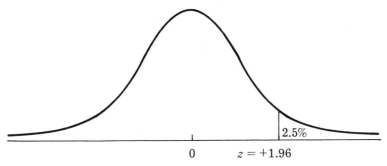

Figure 7.6. Percentage of the normal distribution located beyond a z score of +1.96.

located beyond, or to the right, of the z score +1.96. This proportion may be converted into a percentage by multiplying by 100. Thus, as illustrated in Figure 7.6, 2.5 percent of the normal distribution is located beyond a z score of +1.96. An alternative way of expressing this is that 2.5 percent of the scores in a normal distribution are *more extreme*, in the sense that they are farther from the mean, than a z score equal to +1.96.

It is important to note in this example that the value .0250 that was read from Table C.2 is interpreted as the proportion contained in the *right-hand tail* of the normal curve, because positive z score values are located in the right-hand half of the curve. When dealing with a *negative z* score we will interpret the value obtained from Table C.2 as indicating the proportion of the normal distribution that is located in the *left-hand tail* of the normal curve. Thus 2.5 percent of the normal distribution is also located beyond a z score of −1.96, in the left-hand tail of the curve.

Let us take another example and find the proportion of the normal distribution that is located beyond a z score equal to −0.98. Turning to Table C.2, find the first two digits, 0.9, in the left margin. Then locate the third digit, 8, in the top margin, and read the number in the body of the table at the intersection of this row and column, which in this case is .1635. Converting this proportion into a percentage, we may interpret it as indicating that 16.35 percent of the normal distribution is located beyond a z score of −0.98, as illustrated in Figure 7.7.

Table C.2 can also be used to derive the information presented in Figure 7.3: the percentage of the normal distribution that is located between points along the normal curve. For example, to find the percentage located between the mean and one standard deviation above it, look up a z score value of +1.00 in Table C.2. You will find that 15.87 percent of the distribution is located above that point. Since a total of 50 percent of the distribution is located above the mean, we may determine, by subtracting 15.87 from 50, that 34.13

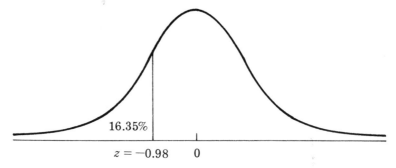

16.35%

$z = -0.98$ 0

Figure 7.7. Percentage of the normal distribution located beyond a z score of -0.98.

percent of the normal distribution is located between the mean and one standard deviation above it. Similarly, according to Table C.2, 2.28 percent of the normal distribution is located above a z score of $+2.00$, leaving 47.72 percent $(50 - 2.28)$ located between the mean and two standard deviations about it. Also, by either adding 34.13 and 2.28 and then subtracting from 50 or subtracting 2.28 from 15.87, we may determine that 13.59 percent of the normal distribution is located between the points that are one and two standard deviations above the mean.

Application of Standard Scores and the Normal Distribution

The main application of z scores and the normal distribution is in inferential statistics and hypothesis testing, which will be discussed in the following chapters. However, these concepts are also very useful for describing and making comparisons within and between distributions of research observations when the shape of the distributions approximate that of the normal curve.

Although, as was mentioned earlier in this chapter, many distributions observed in actual practice are not normal distributions, the z score and normal distribution concepts may be applied in the analysis of distributions that are "approximately normal." While there are statistical tests that are designed to help decide whether the shape of a given distribution is "approximately normal," we will not be concerned with them here. Instead we will make this judgment simply on the basis of visual inspection of the distribution in question. Although this method lacks precision, we do not require a great deal of precision for our present purpose. Furthermore, the requirement of a normal distribution is much less rigid than it may seem at first. This is because the normal distribution is what statisticians refer to as a "robust" concept, meaning that violations of the requirement of a normal distribution have a relatively small effect on the final results of an analysis. While some precision may be sacrificed, much more is gained in terms of the convenience of computations and the interpretability of the results. In general the normal distribution may be applied to the analysis of a distribution with no significant loss of precision as long as the shape of the observed distribution is approximately symmetrical, if not normal. Furthermore the normal distribution may be applied to the analysis of skewed distributions as long as the degree of skew is not extreme. Also, as the sample size increases, the effect in terms of loss of precision in the results tends to decrease. Therefore the shape of a distribution is of less concern for large samples (100 or larger).

Any observed distribution may be transformed into a normal distribution by converting each observation into a z score because, as mentioned earlier, in a normal distribution there is a perfect correspondence between z scores and standard deviation units. For example, converting the mean of 11.6 for Table 7.1, which is derived from Table 6.7, into a z score yields the following result:

$$z = \frac{X - \overline{X}}{\sigma} = \frac{11.6 - 11.6}{7.73} = \frac{0}{7.73} = 0$$

Thus the mean for Table 7.1 has been converted to a z score of 0, which is exactly equal to the mean of the normal distribution. Furthermore a person who travels 19.33 miles is one standard deviation unit above the mean (19.33 = 11.6 + 7.73), and converting 19.33 into a z score we obtain the result

$$z = \frac{X - \overline{X}}{\sigma} = \frac{19.33 - 11.6}{7.73} = \frac{7.73}{7.73} = +1.00$$

Again, this corresponds exactly to the value of a point located one standard deviation unit above the mean in the normal distribution. The reader may wish to verify this relationship for other values; for example, the z score for a person who travels 3.87 miles is equal to −1.00, indicating that the person is one

Table 7.1. Distance to Usual Source of Care

Distance (miles)	f	
0-9	232	$\overline{X} = 11.6$
10-19	204	
20-29	63	$\sigma = 7.73$
30-39	7	
40-49	1	
50-59	1	
	$N = 508$	

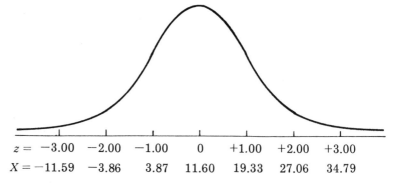

$$z = -3.00 \quad -2.00 \quad -1.00 \quad 0 \quad +1.00 \quad +2.00 \quad +3.00$$
$$X = -11.59 \quad -3.86 \quad 3.87 \quad 11.60 \quad 19.33 \quad 27.06 \quad 34.79$$

Figure 7.8. Relationship between observed distribution values (X) from Table 7.1, z scores, and points along the normal curve.

standard deviation unit below the mean for Table 7.1. Figure 7.8 illustrates the correspondence between values derived from Table 7.1, which are identified as X, and z score values for the normal distribution.

This facilitates comparisons between observations from a single distribution. For example, from Table 7.1, the z score for a person who travels 10 miles is computed as

$$z = \frac{X - \overline{X}}{\sigma} = \frac{10 - 11.6}{7.73} = \frac{-1.6}{7.73} = -0.21$$

and the z score for a person who travels 15 miles is

$$z = \frac{X - \overline{X}}{\sigma} = \frac{15 - 11.6}{7.73} = \frac{3.4}{7.73} = 0.44$$

Looking these z score values up in Table C.2 we find that approximately 41.68 percent of the persons in the distribution travel less than 10 miles. Rounding this percentage to the nearest whole percent, we can express this another way by saying that a person who travels 10 miles is at the 42nd percentile. In comparison, according to Table C.2, approximately 33.00 percent of the persons in the distribution travel more than 15 miles, and by subtracting from 100 we find that 67 percent travel less than 15 miles. Therefore a person who travels 15 miles is at the 67th percentile for this distribution. These results are illustrated in Figure 7.9. Note that percentile rank is determined according to the percentage of the distribution that is below, or to the left, of the score in question. Also, by adding the percentage of persons who travel less than 10 miles to that of persons who travel more than 15 miles ($41.68 + 33 = 74.68$) and subtracting this sum from 100 percent, we determine that 25.32 percent, or approximately one-fourth, of the distribution travel between 10 and 15 miles to their usual source of care.

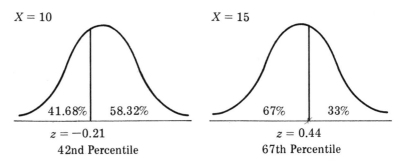

$X = 10$ $X = 15$

41.68% | 58.32%   67% | 33%

$z = -0.21$ $z = 0.44$

42nd Percentile   67th Percentile

Figure 7.9. Comparison of persons traveling 10 and 15 miles to usual source of care, using z scores and the normal distribution.

We may similarly compare observations from two different distributions. For example, we may compare the relative standing of a person who travels 5 miles from the distribution in Table 7.1 (group A) with another person who travels 5 miles but comes from a second distribution (group B) for which the mean is 12.5 and the standard deviation is 4.29. The computation and interpretation of this problem are presented in Figure 7.10, which indicates that a person who travels 5 miles is at the 20th percentile in group A but at only the 4th percentile in group B.

Another application of z scores and the normal distribution is that, given only the mean and standard deviation for a distribution, we may derive a useful estimate of the value of any point in the distribution. By algebraically manipulating the z-score formula (7.1) we may compute the estimated value of any point in an observed distribution according to the following formula:

$$X = z\sigma + \overline{X} \tag{7.2}$$

Group A

$\overline{X} = 11.6$
$\sigma = 7.73$

$z = \dfrac{5 - 11.6}{7.73} = \dfrac{-6.6}{7.73} = -0.85$

Group B

$\overline{X} = 12.5$
$\sigma = 4.29$

$z = \dfrac{5 - 12.5}{4.29} = \dfrac{-7.5}{4.29} = -1.75$

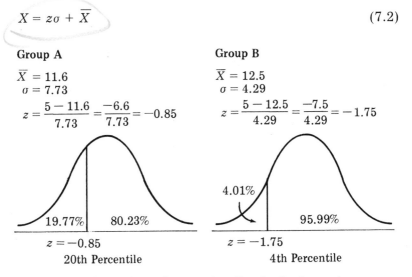

19.77% | 80.23%   4.01%   95.99%

$z = -0.85$ $z = -1.75$

20th Percentile   4th Percentile

Figure 7.10. Comparison of persons traveling 5 miles to usual source of care from two different distributions.

For example, in Table 5.15, the third quartile for the distribution presented in Table 7.1 was computed to be 16.8 miles, indicating that 75 percent of the distribution travel less than 16.8 miles and 25 percent travel more than that distance. Converting the value 16.8 into a z score we obtain the result:

$$z = \frac{X - \overline{X}}{\sigma} = \frac{16.8 - 11.6}{7.73} = \frac{5.20}{7.73} = +0.67$$

Looking up a z score of $+0.67$ in Table C.2 we find that 25.14 percent of the normal distribution is located above this point. Thus a z score of $+0.67$ corresponds to the third quartile in the normal distribution. Instead of using the lengthy interpolation method to compute the third quartile as in Table 5.15, since we know that a z score of $+0.67$ corresponds to the third quartile in the normal distribution, we may substitute this value along with the mean and standard deviation in formula 7.2 and solve for the value of the third quartile, as follows:

$$X = z\sigma + \overline{X} = (+0.67)(7.73) + 11.6 = 5.2 + 11.6 = 16.8$$

We may similarly compute the first quartile for Table 7.1, recognizing that the first quartile for the normal distribution corresponds to a z score of -0.67, because we now wish to divide the distribution at the point where 25 percent of the distribution is below and 75 percent is above. According to formula 7.2 we obtain the result

$$X = z\sigma + \overline{X} = (-0.67)(7.73) + 11.6 = (-5.2) + 11.6 = 6.4$$

While this is not exactly equal to the value of 5.0 which was computed for the first quartile according to the interpolation formula in Table 5.15, it is reasonably close. The slight deviation between these results is due to the fact that the distribution in Table 7.1 is somewhat skewed, which results in a loss of some precision when the conversion to the normal distribution is made.

As a final example, suppose we wish to compute the 80th percentile for Table 7.1. In order to find the z score that corresponds to the 80th percentile in the normal distribution, we look in the body of Table C.2 and locate the proportion value nearest to .2000, because we wish to divide the distribution at the point where 20 percent is above. The value nearest to .2000 in Table C.2 is .2005, which corresponds to a z score of $+0.84$. Using formula 7.2 we may now compute the 80th percentile as

$$X = z\sigma + \overline{X} = (+0.84)(7.73) + 11.6 = 6.5 + 11.6 = 18.1$$

This is almost exactly equal to the value of 18.0 that was computed earlier according to the interpolation formula for Table 5.15.

WORKING WITH AND INTERPRETING DATA

1. Indicate the percentage of the normal distribution that is located both above and below each of the following z score values.

   a. $+1.96$
   b. -1.96
   c. $+1.65$
   d. -1.65
   e. $+1.28$
   f. -1.28
   g. $+2.33$
   h. -2.33

2. Turn back to Chapter 3, question 2, to the data on when members and nonmembers of La Leche League first introduced solid foods into the diet of their first child. Use the z score approach to compute the first quartile and 90th percentile for these distributions. You have already calculated the means and standard deviations for these distributions in Chapter 5, question 1c and Chapter 6, question 1d. Compare your results with your answers for questions 3 and 4 in Chapter 5.

3. If a woman introduced solid foods into her first child's diet at 4 months, what would her percentile ranking be among members and nonmembers of La Leche League? What do these percentile rankings tell you about the distribution of the other women in each group?

4. The mean systolic blood pressure for a group of 300 patients is 125 mm Hg, with a standard deviation equal to 10.2.

   a. What is the z score of a patient who is one and one-half standard deviations *below* the mean?
   b. Compute the interquartile range.
   c. What percentage of the patients have a blood pressure reading of between 100 and 150 mm Hg?
   d. What percentage of the patients have a blood pressure reading of between 125 and 140 mm Hg?
   e. What percentage of the patients have a blood pressure reading of between 110 and 125 mm Hg?

f. What percentage of the patients have a blood pressure reading of higher than 140 mm Hg?

g. What percentage of the patients have a blood pressure reading of below 110 mm Hg?

Inferential Statistics

II

In the previous seven chapters we have considered a wide variety of descriptive statistical techniques. We have stated and applied basic principles for grouping data and presenting them in both tabular and graphic form. In addition simply to grouping data into a series of categories, we considered techniques for representing a distribution of values by calculating a single summary measure, such as the median and the mean. Other measures, such as the range and standard deviation, described the amount of diversity or variation in a distribution of scores. So far we have limited our descriptions, and our conclusions regarding the data, to subjects from whom we had collected some information. For example, in working with the La Leche League data, we used a variety of tables, graphs, and charts to summarize these data and uncover patterns or trends. Our descriptions focused on the total sample of 900 subjects or the subsample of 75 subjects.

On a commonsense level, limiting one's descriptions to the data at hand seems an entirely sensible thing to do. We might reasonably wonder, however, if our conclusions apply also to the thousands of La Leche League members who did not fall into our sample. Or we might like to know if La Leche League members manage their breast-feeding experiences in an appreciably different manner from women who are not affiliated with the organization. Is it possible to generalize beyond one's data? Isn't it going out on a limb to do so? The answer to both these questions is yes. Researchers usually do want to go beyond their data in drawing conclusions about their findings. Such generalization is possible and desirable. On the other hand, generalization entails some degree of sticking one's neck out. This is because one never knows for certain if inferences, generalizations beyond the data, are correct. When researchers use statistical techniques to make generalizations that go beyond their data, they are using statistics differently from the way we have so far in this book. Instead of describing data, they are making inferences from their data.

Interestingly, descriptive and inferential statistics draw on many of the same techniques. For example, depending on the specific inferential technique being employed, we may find ourselves computing a measure of central tendency or dispersion or casting the data into a cross-classification table. Such procedures will no longer be the endpoint of our analysis, however. Rather, they will constitute one of the steps we need to complete before we can make generalizations beyond the data with which we are working. In this chapter we introduce the terms and logic underlying inferential statistics.

Specifically, we introduce the reader to the following: samples, types of hypotheses, sampling distributions, level of significance, inference decisions, and types I and II errors. In Chapter 9 we will show how these concepts are applied in hypothesis testing.

In general the use of inferential statistics makes it possible for the researcher to know how far out on a limb he or she is going when generalizing from a sample to the larger population from which the sample was drawn. The researcher will never be absolutely, 100 percent sure that his or her inferential conclusion is correct. By applying an appropriate inferential statistical technique, however, the researcher can compute the probability that his or her inferential conclusion is correct.

Populations, Samples, and Inference

It is usually necessary to generalize findings because it is usually impossible to collect data from all relevant subjects. To collect data from over 20,000 La Leche League members would have been practically and financially difficult, if not impossible. Similarly, a researcher interested in health needs of rural Americans would probably not have the resources to study *all* rural Americans. Usually researchers collect data from only a portion, often a very small portion, of the subjects in whom they are interested. The process by which a researcher selects research subjects from the pool of all possible subjects is called *sampling*. The larger pool from which sample subjects are drawn is called the *population*. All inferential statistical tests are based on the assumption that the sample data accurately represent the population.

Table 8.1, reproduced from Chapter 3, demonstrates the relationship between inferential statistics and sampling. As pointed out in the discussion of cross-classification tables in Chapter 3, researchers sometimes construct such tables to help them determine if a relationship exists between two variables or if two groups differ from one another with regard to a specific characteristic. Accordingly Table 8.1 has been constructed to shed light on the question "Is duration of breast-

Table 8.1. Cross-Classification of Duration of Breast-Feeding Experience by La Leche League Membership

	Months					
Membership	0–5	6–11	12–17	18–23	Total (%)	N
Yes	7	21	37	35	100	100
No	30	62	8	0	100	50

feeding related to membership in La Leche League?" or "Do members of La Leche League differ from nonmembers with regard to how long they breast-feed their children?" If we are interested in answering this question only as it applies to the 150 subjects shown in the table, we can do so simply by visual examination of the table. Such inspection reveals that differences do exist between members and nonmembers. Comparatively more members fall into the two highest duration categories; comparatively more nonmembers fall into the two lowest duration categories. For this particular sample of 150 cases, a relationship exists between membership and duration of breast-feeding experience. The two groups, member and nonmember, differ from one another.

One might refer to this as a descriptive conclusion, since it is based on the 150 subjects from whom the researchers have collected data. The various descriptive statistical techniques we have considered facilitate making such conclusions. Inferential conclusions, on the other hand, apply not only to the research subjects but to the population from which the sample subjects were selected. Just as descriptive statistics facilitate descriptive conclusions about data, inferential statistics makes it possible for the researcher to reach conclusions about the population(s) from which the sample(s) is drawn. For example, by applying the appropriate inferential statistical techniques to Table 8.1 it is possible to determine if the differences we have observed in these two samples (a sample of 100 members and a sample of 50 nonmembers) provide sufficient evidence to conclude that the *population* of La Leche League members breast-feed longer than the *population* of nonmembers. Before applying an inferential statistical technique to his or her data, the researcher wants to be reasonably certain that those data accurately represent the population from which they were drawn. He or she does this by selecting subjects using a process called probability sampling. Consequently we will begin our discussion of inferential statistics with a brief overview of the characteristics of a probability sample.

While laypersons often are familiar with the term *random sample*, they frequently have an inaccurate view of the characteristics of such a sample. This is because in lay terminology the word random connotes a haphazard or impetuous course of action. As we shall see, random sampling is far from a haphazard process.

In actuality a *simple* random sample is one of several options open to the researcher who is planning to carry out a probability sample. Other possibilities frequently encountered in the nursing research literature are *stratified* and *systematic* sampling. We will not delve into the specifics of these techniques. Nonetheless it is important to remember that all probability sampling techniques are based on characteristically inflexible procedural rules. In general, probability samples conform to the following principles:

1. Every observation in the population has an *equal or known* chance of entering the sample.
2. Every observation included in the sample must be chosen *independently* of every other observation.

The dependence of inferential statistical techniques on probability samples derives from the nature of the inferential conclusions. Remember, these conclusions entail generalizing sample results to the population from which the sample was drawn. Such generalization is justified only if we can be reasonably certain that the sample accurately represents the population from which it was selected. It is important to remember that there are many possible outcomes when a sample of a certain size is drawn from a population. For example, a researcher could have 500 subjects in a population and draw a sample of 50 subjects. If the researcher returned these 50 subjects to the population and picked another sample of 50, it is very unlikely that she or he would select the same 50 persons a second time. The two samples would probably differ. If the researcher continued to draw successive samples of 50 and then returned them to the population, she or he would eventually select many different samples.

Now let's assume that, for each of the samples drawn, the researcher calculates a mean age. Because each sample contains different subjects, we would expect a different mean age for each sample. Because each sample was drawn from the same population, however, we would expect that most of the time these differences would be small. In addition we would expect that the sample means would usually be close to the population mean. Occasionally, due to chance combinations of individuals whose age is atypical, we would come up with large differences, and the sample mean would not accurately represent the population mean. But not only would such occurrences be rare, we would be able to calculate the probability of their occurrence as long as we had sampled using *probability sampling* techniques. This is the reason researchers must use probability sampling techniques if they plan to apply inferential statistical tests to their data.

Moreover, the logic of hypothesis testing assumes that sample results will be compared with certain theoretical populations. The researcher asks, "What is the probability that my sample data were selected from a population with certain specified characteristics?" Using the sample data from Table 8.1 we would ask, "What is the probability of observing differences of this magnitude between members and nonmembers, if the true situation in the populations from which these two samples were drawn is that there is *no* difference between the two groups regarding the duration of their breast-feeding experiences?" (Note that we ask a question about the *opposite* of what we hope to show is true. The logic of this is explained under the discussion of *null hypothesis* later in this chapter.) We will discuss at length the process of comparing sample results with theoretical or hypothetical populations as we consider the steps involved in hypothesis testing. At this point, however, you should simply note that *all* statistical tests assume that the researcher has obtained his or her data through probability sampling.

Research Hypothesis and Null Hypothesis

A hypothesis is a statement of a relationship between variables. Table 8.1 contains two variables, (1) membership and (2) duration of breast-feeding experience. The membership variable has been divided into two categories, member and nonmember. The duration variable has been divided into four categories, 0–5, 6–11, 12–17, and 18–23 months. Even *before* the data were collected we could have stated a hypothesis describing the *expected* relationship between variables in several ways. For example:

1. Members and nonmembers will differ in the duration of their breast-feeding experiences.
2. Members will breast-feed longer than nonmembers.
3. Nonmembers will breast-feed longer than members.
4. Members and nonmembers will not differ in the duration of their breast-feeding experiences.

The first three statements are examples of *research* hypotheses. The fourth statement is a *null* hypothesis. Researchers state their hypotheses *prior* to collecting their data. It is important to remember that these hypotheses refer to the population from which we selected our sample and not to the sample itself.

Research Hypothesis

The researcher's prediction of a certain outcome, what he or she expects to occur, is called the *research hypothesis.* As evidenced in the examples just listed, research hypotheses predict that some sort of difference exists between the groups studied or that a relationship exists between or among the variables being researched. Researchers typically conduct studies because they believe such differences or relationships exist. Research hypotheses can be either *nondirectional* or *directional.* A nondirectional hypothesis predicts only that the variables will be related or the groups under study differ in some way. It says nothing about the nature of the relationship or the difference. Statement 1 of the four hypotheses just listed is an example of a *nondirectional hypothesis*. In contrast a *directional* hypothesis specifies the nature of the relationship or difference. For example, it says that one group scores higher (or lower) than another group or that there is a positive (or negative) relationship between variables. Statements 2 and 3 are examples of directional hypotheses.

Whether a researcher states a directional or a nondirectional research hypothesis depends on the state of knowledge in the area under investigation. To state a nondirectional hypothesis the researcher must believe only that a difference or a relationship exists. The researcher is unable to specify how groups of subjects differ or how variables are related. If the researcher believes he or she knows enough about the subject matter to predict how the groups being studied differ or how the variables are related, he or she states a directional hypothesis. As we shall see, directional hypotheses are always easier to support than nondirectional ones. Therefore, researchers generally prefer to state directional research hypotheses. They are justified in doing so, however, only when previous findings or clinical experience support a directional statement. Whether directional or nondirectional, the research hypothesis is symbolized H_1, H_2, etc., depending on the number of hypotheses being tested.

Null Hypothesis

In contrast to the research hypothesis the null hypothesis is a statement of *no relationship* or *no difference* between groups. Inferential statistical tests are formulated to test null hypotheses like statement 4, which says that members and nonmembers will not differ in the duration of their breast-feeding experiences. The null hypothesis is symbolized H_0.

It is important to remember that a statistical test of a hypothesis is *always* a test of the null hypothesis and that the resulting inference decision will be either to reject or accept the null hypothesis. *We test the null hypothesis by finding out how probable or likely our data are if the null hypothesis is true.* As we shall later discuss, there are statistical tables that allow us to determine what this probability is. For example, by applying an appropriate statistical test to Table 8.1 we can determine the probability of obtaining differences between our samples as large as those observed in Table 8.1 when the populations of members and nonmembers *do not* differ in the duration of their breast-feeding experiences. If this probability is very small; if our data as depicted in Table 8.1 are highly improbable when the null hypothesis is true; then we *reject* the null hypothesis in favor of the research hypothesis. If the research results are quite probable, then we *accept* the null hypothesis. The decision to accept or reject the null hypothesis is called the *inference decision*. The decision is inferential because it refers to the population from which we selected our sample subjects. As previously stated, inferential statistical tests make it possible to reach conclusions about populations based on a sample of the population. We use a sample to make inferences about a population.

The null hypothesis is a statement of either no difference between groups or no relationship between variables. The research hypothesis, as we have discussed, is a statement that a difference or a relationship exists. Therefore, when we reject the null hypothesis, we accept the research hypothesis; when we accept the null hypothesis, we reject the research hypothesis. In short we take the *opposite* action on these two kinds of hypotheses. Rejecting the null hypothesis implies accepting the research hypothesis and vice versa. As stated in the previous discussion, our decision to accept or reject the null hypothesis hinges on the probability of obtaining the research results *if the null hypothesis is true.* Two questions remain:

1. How improbable must the results be before we can reject the null hypothesis?
2. How do we determine the probability of the research results if the null hypothesis is true?

In order to answer the first question one has to understand something called *level of significance.* To answer the second question one has to do the following:

1. Calculate a standardized score.
2. Use the appropriate probability table to find the probability of obtaining the calculated standardized score when the null hypothesis is *true.*

Level of Significance

In the previous section we stated that we can reject the null hypothesis when the sample data are very unlikely to occur if the null hypothesis is true. There is a conventional statistical definition of "very unlikely," called *level of significance.* The level of significance is the cut-off point at which probability is small enough that we are able to *reject* the null hypothesis.[1] Nursing, like other disciplines, commonly uses two levels of significance, .05 and .01, with .05 being used more often. When a researcher reports results as significant at the .05 level, we can expect the sample result to occur 5 percent of the time (five times in every 100 samples) if H_0 is true. A researcher who states that results are significant at the .01 level is saying

---

[1] This critical value along a sampling distribution is also referred to as the *alpha level* and is symbolized by the lowercase Greek letter α.

that the sample result would occur 1 percent of the time (once in every 100 samples) if H_0 were true. When the researcher speaks of results as significant, it means he or she has *rejected* the null hypothesis in favor of the research hypothesis. Having collected data from a probability sample of subjects, we calculate the probability of getting our specific results when the null hypothesis is *true*. If we have decided to use the .05 level of significance and this probability is .05 or less, we *reject* the null hypothesis. For example, the null hypothesis associated with Table 8.1 is that members and nonmembers will not differ in the duration of their breast-feeding experiences. By applying a statistical test to Table 8.1 we can find the probability of getting this table if this null hypothesis is true. If this probability is .05 or less, we reject the null hypothesis in favor of whatever research hypothesis we have stated. When we reject the null hypothesis, we say our results are significant; thus the term *level of significance*.

In order to make the inference decision to accept or reject the null hypothesis at a specific level of significance, we need to know the probability of obtaining the sample results if the null hypothesis is true. We find this probability by first converting our data to a standardized score and then using a sampling distribution to find the probability of obtaining that standardized score when the null hypothesis is true.

Standardized Scores and Sampling Distributions

You were introduced to both concepts—standardized scores and sampling distributions—when you calculated a z score in Chapter 7. A z score is one kind of standardized score. Others with which we will deal include the chi-square score, t score, and Mann-Whitney U score. We will also discuss how to convert a variety of statistics into z scores and how to use z scores to test a null hypothesis.

By converting sets of data into standardized scores we are able to make use of known sampling distributions to determine the probability of our results. A *sampling distribution* is a special kind of frequency distribution. It depicts a series of standardized scores and the probabilities associated with each score when the null hypothesis is true. In other words it reflects the *distribution* of standardized scores obtained by converting *sample* data into standardized scores. Each such score in the sampling distribution has an associated probability. This is the probability of obtaining a certain standardized score or a more extreme one if the null hypothesis is true. If the probability of the standardized score is *equal to* or *less than* what the researcher has set as his or her level of significance, then the researcher can *reject* the null hypothesis. Sampling distributions are summarized in the form of probability tables such as the normal curve table. The other standardized scores that we will discuss also have sampling distributions that are summarized in probability tables. These tables are constructed in a number of different ways, and we will discuss how to use the different tables as we present various standardized scores in the following chapters. Since you are already familiar with z scores and the normal curve probability table, we will use these here to illustrate the concepts we have been discussing.

For example, we might take a raw score of 85 on an examination and find that it converts to a z score of 1.00. Using the normal probability curve we would determine that there is about a 16 percent probability that a z score of 1.00 would be exceeded. With a probability of .16 (16 %) it would not be possible to reject a null hypothesis at the .05 level of significance. To reject the null hypothesis our data would have to convert to a z score that would be exceeded 5 percent of the time or less. Remember, all probability tables summarize sampling distributions. Think of these tables as curves filled with standardized scores, some of which are much more likely than others to occur if the null hypothesis is true. The more probable standardized scores fall near the center of the curve. The less probable standardized scores fall in the tails of the curve. Standardized scores falling close to the center of the curve will be smaller in magnitude than those falling in the tails. Thus, as a standardized score *increases* in size, the probability of the score *decreases.*

If the standardized score is large enough to allow the researcher to reject the null hypothesis, it is said to lie within the *region of rejection* of the curve depicting the sampling distribution of standardized scores. The size of the region of rejection depends on the level of significance. When the level of significance is .05, the region of rejection makes up 5 percent of the curve. When the level of significance is .01, the region of rejection makes up 1 percent of the curve. The region of rejection is always located in the tail or tails of the curve. Its location varies depending on whether or not the research hypothesis is directional or nondirectional. When the research hypothesis is directional, the entire region of rejection is located in *either* the upper (right-hand) *or* the lower (left-hand) tail of the curve. When the research hypothesis is nondirectional, the region of rejection is *equally* divided between the upper and lower tails of the curve. Figure 8.1 illustrates these possibilities. It is apparent from the figure why directional hypotheses are also referred to as *one-tailed* and nondirectional hypotheses are also referred to as *two-tailed.*

The standardized score needed to reject the null hypothesis will vary depending on which statistical test is being applied to the data and whether the research hypothesis is directional or nondirectional. Using the familiar z score as an example, we see by referring to Table C.2 that the z scores

.05 Level of significance—directional hypothesis

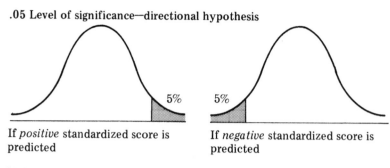

5%   5%

If *positive* standardized score is
predicted

If *negative* standardized score is
predicted

.05 Level of significance—nondirectional hypothesis

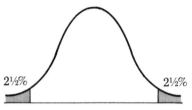

2½%   2½%

Figure 8.1. Region of rejection (*shaded area*) and directional and
nondirectional hypotheses.

that correspond to the .05 level of significance when a nondirectional hypothesis has been stated are $+1.96$ and -1.96.
In terms of absolute value 1.96 is the smallest z score the researcher can calculate and still have results significant at the
.05 level when the research hypothesis is nondirectional. The
minimum z score needed for significance at the .05 level
when a directional hypothesis has been stated is ± 1.65. Figure 8.2 pictures this situation. As can be seen in this figure,
it takes a smaller standardized score to reject the null hypothesis when one has stated a *directional* hypothesis. Thus it is
comparatively *easier* to reject the null hypothesis if one has
stated a directional hypothesis. Remember that if you calculate a standardized score that falls into the region of rejection, the null hypothesis is *rejected.* If you calculate a
standardized score that falls outside the region of rejection,
the null hypothesis is *accepted.* Sometimes the region of
rejection is entirely located in one tail of the probability
curve; sometimes it is evenly divided between the two tails
of the curve. The research hypothesis determines the *location*
of the region of rejection. The level of significance determines the *size* of the region of rejection. Our inference decision is to reject the null hypothesis when the standardized
score falls within the region of rejection. Our inference decision is to accept the null hypothesis when the standardized
score falls outside the region of rejection.

Inference Decisions and Type I and Type II Errors

Hypothesis testing is always a "sporting proposition," since
one is never certain if one's inference decision is correct. One

Nondirectional hypothesis

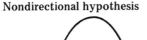
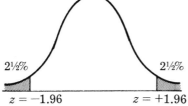

$z = -1.96$ ⠀⠀⠀ $z = +1.96$

2½% ⠀⠀⠀ 2½%

Directional hypothesis

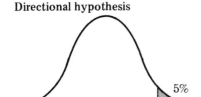
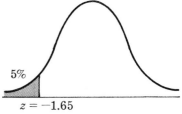

5% ⠀⠀⠀ 5%

$z = +1.65$ ⠀⠀⠀ $z = -1.65$

When *positive* standardized score is predicted ⠀⠀⠀ When *negative* standardized score is predicted

Figure 8.2. Region of rejection at .05 level of significance when re-searcher has stated a *nondirectional* and a *directional* hypothesis.

only knows the *probability* of its being incorrect. When we reject the null hypothesis at the .05 level of significance, there is a 5 percent chance that we have made an incorrect decision. There is a 5 percent chance of obtaining a sample result even if the null hypothesis is true for the population. In other words, one can be only 95 percent confident that the decision made is the correct one. One can never be 100 percent confident of making the correct decision in rejecting the null hypothesis. No matter how large the standardized score, there is still a small probability that the null hypothesis is correct. Thus it is impossible to completely prove or disprove a hypothesis using statistics.

Similarly, one never knows for certain if one is correct in accepting a null hypothesis. For example, if we calculate a standardized score with an associated probability of .15, and our level of significance is .05, we would accept the null hypothesis. In accepting H_0 we could be wrong 85 percent of the time, since there is only a 15 percent probability of obtaining the sample result when the null hypothesis is true. As you can see, it is more difficult to reject a null hypothesis than to accept it. This means that researchers generally have to have rather convincing evidence before they can reject the null hypothesis in favor of the research hypothesis they are hoping to support.

If the null hypothesis is false and we reject it, or if it is true and we accept it, we have made a correct decision. On the other hand, if we reject a true null hypothesis or accept a false null hypothesis, we have made an incorrect decision.

142

These two kinds of errors are called *type I* (alpha) and *type II* (beta) errors.

We have made a type I error if we reject a true null hypothesis. This is the type of error we make if we conclude that the sample data indicate that a difference or a relationship exists when this is not the case for the population from which the sample was drawn. We make a type I error when we are wrong in *rejecting* the null hypothesis. Thus, whenever a researcher rejects the null hypothesis, he or she is risking a type I error. The probability of making such an error equals the level of significance. If we reject the null hypothesis at the .05 level of significance, we have a 5 percent chance of making a type I error. If we reject the null hypothesis at the .01 level of significance, we have a 1 percent chance of making a type I error. Thus, as the level of significance moves from .05 to .01, there is less probability of making a type I error. Type I errors are symbolized by the lowercase of the Greek letter alpha (α) and are therefore often referred to as *alpha errors*.

We have made a type II error if we accept a false null hypothesis. This is the type of error we make if we conclude that the sample data indicate that no significant difference or relationship exists when this is not the case for the population from which the sample was drawn. We make a type II error when we are wrong in *accepting* the null hypothesis. Thus, whenever a researcher accepts the null hypothesis, he or she is risking a type II error. The maximum probability of making a type II error equals 1 minus the probability of the standardized score we have calculated. Accordingly, if the probability associated with a result is .20, there is as much as an 80 percent probability of making a type II error if the null hypothesis is accepted. Type II errors are symbolized by the lowercase of the Greek letter beta (β) and are therefore often referred to as *beta errors*. Neither the researcher nor the reader knows for certain if a correct or incorrect inference decision has been made. What is known is the probability of the decision being incorrect and the type of decision error being risked. This situation is summarized below.

	Situation in population	
Inference decision	H_0 *true*	H_0 *false*
Reject H_0	Type I error	Correct decision
Accept H_0	Correct decision	Type II error

In sum, inferential statistical procedures provide a standardized way for determining the probability that differences or relationships observed in a sample are likely to occur in the population as well. Any researcher looking at the same data and using the same level of significance would reach the same decision. In other words, the decision is completely objective.

143   The word *significant* has a very precise meaning when used in statistics. It refers to the probability associated with the research findings. For example, if the findings would occur 5 percent of the time or less when the null hypothesis is true, the results are called significant. This is *statistical significance*. Statistical significance is not a guarantee that results are clinically significant or relevant, however. It is possible for a set of results to be statistically significant but have little or no *substantive significance*. The determination of statistical significance is a highly systematized and objective process. The evaluation of the practical or substantive significance of a set of data is a much more subjective process. It depends on your own assessment of the overall quality of the research as well as the applicability of the results to your own particular setting or situation. Obviously this evaluation will vary from person to person. Statistical tests of significance are invaluable aids to the analysis of a set of data. However, they must be interpreted within the context of the entire study and according to the consumer's purposes in reading a study or the researcher's purposes for reporting it.

WORKING WITH AND INTERPRETING DATA

1. Answer the following on the basis of Lindeman and Van Aernam's study, Nursing intervention with the presurgical patient: Effects of structured and unstructured preoperative teaching. *Nursing Research* 20:319–332, 1971.

   a. What are the authors' research hypotheses?
   b. Are these hypotheses directional or nondirectional?
   c. Restate each research hypothesis in the form of a null hypothesis.
   d. Assuming the authors set their level of significance at .05, what was their inference decision with regard to each null hypothesis?
   e. For each inference decision, indicate whether the authors were risking a type I or type II error.
   f. On the basis of these findings, what is the probability that both patients who receive structured preoperative teaching and those who do not will have the same expiratory flow rate scores?

2. Answer the following on the basis of Keck and Walther's study, Nurse encounters with dying and non-dying patients. *Nursing Research* 26:465–469, 1977.

   The authors' research is based on the following questions:

   Do nurses differ in the amount of time they spend with dying and nondying patients?

Do nurses differ in the amount of verbal communication they have with dying and nondying patients?

a. Restate the first research question in the form of a *nondirectional* research hypothesis.
b. Restate the second research question in the form of a *directional* research hypothesis.
c. Restate either research question in the form of a null hypothesis.
d. With regard to the first question, the authors report that their results were significant at the .004 level of probability. Assuming they set their level of significance at .05, what would their inference decision be for the null hypothesis?
e. In making this inference decision were the authors risking a type I or a type II error?
f. The authors report that they accepted the null hypothesis with regard to the second question. What does this tell us about the amount of verbal communication that nurses have with dying and nondying patients?

Hypothesis Testing with Nominal Level Data

In the previous chapter we considered the concepts that underlie hypothesis testing. In this chapter we will learn to apply these concepts by following a series of seven steps:

1. State a research hypothesis.
2. State a null hypothesis.
3. Set a level of significance.
4. Determine what sampling distribution will be used to find the probability of the result(s) when the null hypothesis is true.
5. Specify the region of rejection and the minimum standardized score needed for the result(s) to be significant.
6. Convert the data into a standardized score.
7. Make an inference decision regarding the null hypothesis.

These steps constitute a fixed order, a standard procedure that is always followed in making a statistical test of a hypothesis. While the steps do not vary, the specific statistical test applied to the data does. In this and the next two chapters we will consider a variety of statistical techniques for converting raw data to standardized scores. These standardized scores will, in turn, be interpreted using a variety of sampling distributions. These sampling distributions are presented in the form of probability tables in Appendix C of this book. For each statistical technique we apply to a set of raw data, we will go through the above seven steps to test a hypothesis. Eventually the process should become routine, even second nature.

Throughout the discussion we will concentrate on selecting an appropriate statistical technique for testing a given null hypothesis. All statistical tests have specific requirements regarding their application. For example, some can only be applied to interval level data, while others can be used with ordinal or nominal data. Some statistics make assumptions about the nature of the population from which the sample was selected; others do not. The researcher must take these requirements into account in choosing a statistical test. The test chosen must be appropriate for the kind of data collected. Failure to match the statistical test to the data leads to misleading or meaningless results. The situation is analogous to that of choosing an appropriate measure of central tendency. We know that in order to calculate a mean, we must have interval level data: to calculate a mean with nominal data is meaningless. Also, the mean will be misleading if the data set includes any extremely low or extremely high scores.

In addition, the original research question influences the choice of a statistical test. For example, even though two researchers have both collected interval level data, they will not necessarily apply the same statistical test to the data. One researcher may be asking, "Is there a *difference* between groups A and B?" The other is asking, "Are variables X and Y *related*?" Certain statistics test for differences between or among groups of observations or subjects; others evaluate the nature of the relationship between or among variables. In this and the following two chapters we will look at a variety of techniques for determining whether two or more groups significantly *differ* from one another. The tests have been divided with regard to level of measurement. This chapter describes techniques appropriate for nominal level data. Chapter 10 looks at techniques most often applied to ordinal level data, and Chapter 11 presents statistical tests applied to interval level data.

Chi-Square: An Example and Overview

Chi-square (symbolized χ^2) is a statistical test commonly used when the researcher has nominal level data and wants to determine if two or more groups differ in some respect. Table 9.1 is an example of such a situation. As pointed out in Chapter 3, researchers sometimes construct such tables to shed light on questions like "Do La Leche League members differ from nonmembers with regard to how long they breastfeed their children?" By applying the chi-square statistical test to these data, it will be possible to determine the probability that the differences between these two random *samples* of members and nonmembers reflect corresponding differences in the *populations* from which they were selected.

Chi-square is another example of a standardized score. In the following section we will go through the steps necessary to convert the data in Table 9.1 to a chi-square score. Then, to determine the probability of getting this particular score when the null hypothesis is *true*, we will refer to a chi-square probability table. If the probability associated with the chi-square score we have calculated is .05 or less, we will reject the null

Table 9.1. Duration of Breast-Feeding Experience by La Leche League Membership

	Duration		
Membership	*< 12 months*	*≥ 12 months*	*Total*
Yes	28	72	100
No	32	18	50
Total	60	90	$N = 150$

hypothesis in favor of the research hypothesis. In terms of this specific example, by converting our raw data to a chi-square score, we will be able to find the probability that the observed differences between the member and nonmember samples hold for the populations from which they were randomly selected.

In applying the chi-square statistical test to Table 9.1, we will go through the series of seven steps (listed at the beginning of this chapter) that must be followed in any statistical test of a hypothesis. Since this is the first time we have actually applied these steps, we will briefly review and explain the content of each one.

Step 1: State a research hypothesis (H_1). H_1 is stated as follows: There is a difference between La Leche League members and nonmembers with regard to how long they breast-feed their children.

Note that this is a nondirectional research hypothesis. It does not predict which of the two groups will breast-feed for the longer time span. Although the researcher might feel justified in making a directional prediction, the chi-square test is not sensitive to the way in which groups differ. Because of the way it is calculated, chi-square is always a positive number and will always be located in the positive or right-hand tail of the curve. In order to state a directional research hypothesis, however, we must be working with a statistical test that can take on both positive and negative values and thereby reflect the nature of the difference between or among groups. Therefore a nondirectional research hypothesis must *always* be stated for the chi-square test.

Step 2: State a null hypothesis (H_0). As always, the null hypothesis in this case is a statement of no difference between the two groups being studied.

H_0 is stated as follows: There is no difference between La Leche League members and nonmembers with regard to how long they breast-feed their children.

Step 3: Set a level of significance (α). We will use the conventional level of significance of .05. Thus, if the probability of obtaining Table 9.1 when the null hypothesis is true is .05 or less, we will *reject* the null hypothesis. We could also have set our level of significance at .01. Since .05 and .01 are conventionally used levels of significance, there is no need for the researcher to explain or justify his or her choice of either of these. However, if the researcher breaks with convention and decides to use some other level of significance, for example .10 or .001, he or she should explain to the reader the reason for this break with tradition. Researchers engaged in exploratory research sometimes set their level of significance above the .05 level of probability. They justify this in terms of not wanting to inhibit further research in a relatively unexplored area simply because results were not significant at the .05 level. On the other hand, investigators whose findings are likely to be applied in "life and death" situations are inclined to lower the probability needed for rejecting the null hypothesis and thus decrease the probability of making a type I error.

Step 4: Determine what sampling distribution will be used to find the probability of the results when the null hypothesis is true. In the present case we will use the chi-square distribution, as summarized in Table C.3 of the Appendix. Table C.3 gives the probability of calculating specific chi-square values when the null hypothesis is true. The numbers in the body of the table are the *minimum* chi-square values needed to reject the null hypothesis at a given level of significance. We will discuss how this table is used under step 5. We have decided to use a chi-square test because of the nature of our research hypothesis and our data. Whenever we have nominal or higher level data that can be cast in a cross-classification table for purposes of determining if differences exist between or among sample groups, it is possible to calculate chi-square. (See discussion under Restrictions on the Use of Chi-Square for specific qualifications pertaining to its use.)

Note that it is possible to use chi-square for higher than nominal level data; however, it is usually not the best or most appropriate technique. This is because, by casting the data into discrete categories, the chi-square statistic treats all data as if it were nominal regardless of the level of measurement. This means that when chi-square is applied to ordinal or interval level data, we waste information by not taking full advantage of the measurement properties of the data.

In sum, step 4 entails selecting an appropriate statistical test to apply to the data on the basis of the nature of the research hypothesis and the level at which the data have been measured. Different statistical tests have different sampling distributions. Thus, in selecting a statistical test, the researcher simultaneously selects the sampling distribution to use to find the probability of his or her results when the null hypothesis is true.

Step 5: Specify the region of rejection and the minimum standardized score needed for the results to be significant. In step 5 we pull together the decisions made in the previous steps and literally draw a picture of the situation that will allow us to reject the null hypothesis (Fig. 9.1). The shaded area in Figure 9.1 constitutes 5 percent of the total curve. If we calculate a chi-square score that falls into this portion of the curve, we will *reject* the null hypothesis, hence the shaded portion of the curve is called the *region of rejection*. The pro-

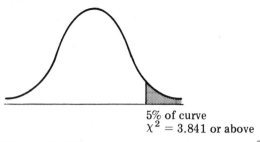

5% of curve
$\chi^2 = 3.841$ or above

Figure 9.1. Region of rejection and minimum χ^2 value needed to reject H_0.*

portion of the curve that makes up the region of rejection is equal in size to whatever level of significance has been established in step 3. If the level of significance is .05, then 5 percent of the curve is set aside as the region of rejection; if the level of significance is .01, then 1 percent of the curve is set aside as the region of rejection. The chi-square value of 3.841 is the minimum chi-square value needed to reject the null hypothesis at the .05 level of significance for a 2 × 2 table. That is, when the null hypothesis is true, we will calculate a chi-square value of 3.841 or greater 5 percent of the time due to the workings of chance in drawing a random sample. Relating this to our specific example, the null hypothesis states there is no difference between La Leche League members and non-members with regard to how long they breast-feed their children. Sampling from a population of members and one of non-members we would get a chi-square score of 3.841 or greater 5 percent of the time, even if there is no difference between these two populations in the length of breast-feeding. This is why hypothesis testing is ultimately a "sporting proposition." If we calculate a chi-square of 3.841 or above in this case, we will reject the null hypothesis. However, for an infinite number of trials we will be wrong in deciding to reject the null hypothesis 5 percent of the time. We will discuss this matter further under step 7.

In order to determine the minimum chi-square score needed to reject the null hypothesis, the reader has to know how to use Table C.3. As we have noted before, this table summarizes the chi-square sampling distribution. Unlike the normal probability distribution, the chi-square distribution is made up of a number of different but related curves. Which curve the researcher uses to find the minimum chi-square value needed to reject the null hypothesis depends on the size of the cross-classification table into which the data have been cast. A table's size is determined by the number of rows and the number of columns it contains. A table with two rows and two columns, like Table 9.1, is a 2 × 2 table. It is customary

*For simplicity, the chi-square curve is pictured here as similar in shape to the normal probability curve. In actuality, it has a somewhat different shape.

to indicate the number of rows first and the number of columns second. In Table C.3 the size of the chi-square table is indicated under the column labeled "df." df stands for *degrees of freedom*. The number of degrees of freedom for any contingency table in which the marginal totals are reported is the number of cells that can be filled in before we automatically know the frequencies in all other cells. Below, Table 9.1 is reproduced listing only the marginal totals.[1]

	Duration		
Membership	*< 12 months*	*≥ 12 months*	*Row total*
Yes	Cell A	Cell B	100
No	Cell C	Cell D	50
Column total	60	90	
		Row and Column total	150

Experimenting on your own, you can see that as soon as you fill in a frequency for any one cell, you can determine the frequencies in the three remaining cells. By using the following formula you can determine the degrees of freedom for any cross-classification table.

$$df = (R - 1)(C - 1)$$

where R = number of rows in the table
C = number of columns in the table

Thus the degrees of freedom for Table 9.1 equal 1 or $[(2-1)(2-1)]$.

To determine the minimum chi-square score needed to reject the null hypothesis at a certain level of significance, the researcher first has to determine the degrees of freedom in his or her cross-classification table. Each row in Table C.3 summarizes a separate chi-square curve. The size of the contingency table with which the researcher is working determines with which row the researcher should be concerned. The level of significance (.05 or .01) set in step 3 determines which column is of interest to the investigator. In the example we are interested in the first row of Table C.3 and the .05 column. The number corresponding to the intersection of these is 3.841. This is the minimum chi-square score needed to reject the null hypothesis. In step 6, we will convert Table 9.1 into a standardized chi-square score and see if this score is large enough to allow us to reject the null hypothesis.

In general, as the size of the cross-classification table and hence the degrees of freedom increase, the size of the minimum chi-square score needed to reject the null hypothesis also increases in size. Also, the size of the chi-square score needed

[1] The cells of tables are conventionally lettered from left to right across the rows.

to reject the null hypothesis is always larger at the .01 than at the .05 level of significance.

In summary, by depicting the region of rejection, we can picture the situation that will allow us to reject the null hypothesis. To do this, we need only to know the level of significance and the minimum standardized score needed to reject the null hypothesis at the stated level of significance. When applying a chi-square test to the data, we need to know the degrees of freedom contained in the contingency table with which we are working. We find this by using the formula $(R - 1)(C - 1)$. Referring to Table C.3 we find the number that corresponds to the intersection of the appropriate degrees of freedom row and level of significance column. The number is the minimum chi-square score needed to reject the null hypothesis. As mentioned before, the region of rejection for chi-square will *always* be located in the positive tail of the curve, since chi-square is always a positive value. The exercises at the end of this chapter provide additional practice in determining degrees of freedom and locating the region of rejection.

Step 6: Convert the data into a standardized score. Step 6 is the technical step of the hypothesis testing process. We now need to convert the data in Table 9.1 into a standardized score. This conversion is accomplished by applying the following formula to the data:

$$\chi^2 = \Sigma \frac{(O-E)^2}{E} \tag{9.1}$$

where O = observed frequency in each cell of the cross-classification table

E = expected frequency in each cell when the null hypothesis is true

The formula entails comparing our data as depicted in the cross-classification table (Table 9.1) with a second, hypothetical, cross-classification table. The second table depicts what frequencies we would expect in each cell if the null hypothesis is true. This second, hypothetical, table of expected frequencies is relatively easy to construct. We begin by again repeating Table 9.1, showing only the marginal totals and labeling the cells A through D.

	Duration		
Membership	*< 12 months*	*≥ 12 months*	*Total*
Yes	A	B	100
No	C	D	50
Total	60	90	$N =$ 150

Note that 40 percent (60/150) of the total sample breast-fed for less than 12 months and 60 percent (90/150) of the total sample breast-fed for 12 months or more. If the null hypothesis is true, we would expect these percentages to hold true for the two membership categories. That is, if there is no difference in duration of breast-feeding between members and nonmembers we would expect that 40 percent of each group would breast-feed for less than 12 months and 60 percent of each group would breast-feed for 12 months or more. In other words, if H_0 is true and there is no difference between members and nonmembers with regard to how long they breast-feed, we would expect the proportion of members and nonmembers breast-feeding for *each* time interval to be equivalent to the proportion of the entire sample that breast-fed for each time interval. In order to find expected frequencies for the less than 12 month time interval we simply calculate 40 percent of each row total. To find expected frequencies for the 12 months or more time interval, we calculate 60 percent of each of these row totals. These calculations yield the following expected frequencies:

< 12 months	*≥ 12 months*
$.40 \times 100 = 40$	$.60 \times 100 = 60$
$.40 \times\ \ 50 = 20$	$.60 \times\ \ 50 = 30$

We would expect twice as many members as nonmembers in each column, because there are twice as many members (100) than nonmembers (50) in the sample.

There is a computational shortcut for calculating expected frequencies. For each cell this is

$$\frac{\text{Row total} \times \text{Column total}}{N}$$

With the computational formula the expected frequency for each cell is calculated as follows:

Cell	Computation of expected frequency
A	$\dfrac{100 \times 60}{150} = 40$
B	$\dfrac{100 \times 90}{150} = 60$
C	$\dfrac{50 \times 60}{150} = 20$
D	$\dfrac{50 \times 90}{150} = 30$

The logic underlying the chi-square test entails a comparison of the observed frequencies with those one would expect to find when the null hypothesis is true. Making this comparison for the present example, we find the following differences between the observed and expected cell frequencies:

Cell	(O) Observed frequency	(E) Expected frequency	(O—E) Difference
A	28	40	−12
B	72	60	12
C	32	20	12
D	18	30	−12
			$\Sigma = 0$

We can see that all the observed scores deviate from what we would expect if the null hypothesis were true. What we need now is some way of summarizing these differences into a single, standardized score. As the Difference column of the comparison indicates, summing the differences between observed and expected scores does not yield a useful standardized score. The sum of these differences will always equal zero. This being the case, we will follow the same procedure we used in calculating the standard deviation, and square each of these difference scores. This squaring process, which is called for in the numerator of the chi-square formula (formula 9.1), $(O—E)^2$, is shown below.

Cell	$(O—E)^2$
A	144
B	144
C	144
D	144

A problem of the squaring process is that it inflates the numbers with which we are working. Therefore, to return the numbers to the context of the original data, we divide each of these squared deviation scores by the expected frequency (E) for each cell. This division process is indicated by the denominator of the chi-square formula,

Cell	$(O—E)^2/E$
A	$\dfrac{144}{40} = 3.6$
B	$\dfrac{144}{60} = 2.4$
C	$\dfrac{144}{20} = 7.2$
D	$\dfrac{144}{30} = 4.8$
	$\Sigma = \quad 18.00$

The final step in calculating chi-square is to sum all the $(O-E)^2/E$ values as indicated by the summation sign (Σ) in the formula. This final step yields a chi-square value of 18.00. This is the standardized score we obtain when we convert Table 9.1 to a chi-square score. The various steps in actually calculating chi-square are shown below.

Calculation of χ^2 Score

Cell	O	E	$O-E$	$(O-E)^2$	$(O-E)^2/E$	χ^2
A	28	40	−12	144	3.6	18.00
B	72	60	12	144	2.4	
C	32	20	12	144	7.2	
D	18	30	−12	144	4.8	

$$\Sigma = 18.00$$

Once we have converted the raw data to a standardized score by calculating a chi-square value, we can make an inference decision regarding the null hypothesis.

Step 7: Make an inference decision regarding the null hypothesis. In deciding whether to accept or reject the null hypothesis (the inference decision) we compare the standardized score calculated in step 6 with the minimum chi-square value needed to reject the null hypothesis. In step 5 we determined this minimum value to be 3.841. Since the chi-square value of 18.00 that we have calculated is *larger* than the minimum value needed to reject the null hypothesis, our inference decision is to reject the null hypothesis in favor of the research hypothesis. Pictorially we can see that a chi-square value of 18.00 clearly falls into the shaded portion of the curve in Figure 9.1; that is, 18.00 is in the region of rejection for the sampling distribution of chi-square that corresponds to a cross-classification table with 1 degree of freedom.

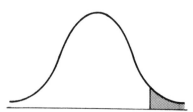

5% of curve containing χ^2 values of 3.841 and above

Furthermore, since our chi-square value of 18.00 is larger than the minimum chi-square value of 6.635 needed to reject the null hypothesis at the .01 level, we can conclude that our results are significant at the .01 level. Two things are important to remember about the decision to reject the null hypothesis. First, the decision is an *inference* decision; it refers to the *populations* of members and nonmembers and not to the data depicted in Table 9.1. Second, we have only *rejected* the null hypothesis, we have not *disproved* it. We still don't know if the null hypothesis is true or false. *We do know that the probability of getting Table 9.1 is less than 1 percent if the null hypothesis is true,* thus lending support to our research hypothesis. Since we have rejected the null hypothesis, we are risking a type I or alpha error. We are in danger of rejecting a null hypothesis that is true. There is no way of knowing if we have committed a type I error. We only know that this is the type of error we are risking and that the probability of making it is less than 1 percent, since our results are significant at the .01 level.

In deciding to reject the null hypothesis, we have completed the final step in testing the null hypothesis. To summarize the seven steps we have followed:

1. H_1 : There is a difference between La Leche League members and nonmembers with regard to how long they breast-feed their children.
2. H_0 : There is no difference between La Leche League members and nonmembers with regard to how long they breast-feed their children.
3. Level of significance: .05.
4. Sampling distribution: The chi-square distribution corresponding to a cross-classification table with one degree of freedom.
5. Region of rejection and minimum standardized score needed for results to be significant:

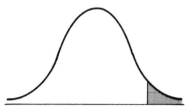

3.841 = Minimum χ^2 value needed to reject H_0 when df = 1

6. Computation of standardized score: $\chi^2 = \Sigma \dfrac{(O-E)^2}{E}$
   = 18.00.
7. Inference decision: Reject H_0.

Reporting and Evaluating Chi-Square

Researchers applying a chi-square test to their data will report it in a table similar to Table 9.2. Note that percentages are presented in the cells of the table to facilitate comparisons between members and nonmembers.

Table 9.2. Duration of Breast-Feeding Experience by La Leche League Membership

Membership	Duration		Total	n
	< 12 months	≥ 12 months		
Yes	28	72	100	100
No	64	36	100	50

$\chi^2 = 18.00$
df = 1
$p < .01$

They should also discuss their findings in a "Results" section of their article: for example,

The data yielded a chi-square value of 18.00, which is significant beyond the .01 level of significance. Thus the findings of this study indicate that La Leche League members breast-feed their children for a longer duration of time than nonmembers.

Having summarized the findings, the researcher would probably go on to discuss why he or she believes these group differences occur. Finally, it is important to keep in mind that the chi-square test does not indicate the direction or strength of the relationship between the variables under study. It tells us only the probability that a relationship exists. This will be discussed further in Chapter 12, when measures of association are introduced.

Restrictions on the Use of Chi-Square

In addition to being able to test hypotheses using the chi-square test and to understand this test when it is presented in the literature, one also needs to know when chi-square has been appropriately applied and when it has not been. Under step 4 we discussed some general requirements for the use of chi-square. At that point we noted that whenever we have nominal or higher level data that can be cast in a cross-classification table for purposes of determining if differences exist between or among sample groups, it is possible to calculate chi-square. There are several restrictions on the application of chi-square, as follows:

1. Do not calculate chi-square on a percentage table. Percentage values must first be converted to raw frequencies.
2. Do not calculate chi-square if *any expected frequency* is zero.
3. Do not calculate chi-square if more than 20 percent of the *expected frequencies* are less than 5.

4. Do not calculate chi-square for a 2×2 table having any expected frequency between 5 and 10 without applying a Yates Correction for continuity to the calculations.

All these restrictions stem from the fact that the chi-square test is quite sensitive to sample size. In general, as the sample size gets larger, it becomes *easier* to reject the null hypothesis when using chi-square. If we were to calculate chi-square using a percentage table, our N would be 100, because the table would total to 100 percent. However, if our actual sample consisted of less than 100 individuals we would be increasing (unfairly) our chances of rejecting the null hypothesis. On the other hand, if there were more than 100 individuals in our sample, we would be decreasing our chances of rejecting the null hypothesis. To apply a chi-square test to a percentage table, it is necessary first to convert the percentages to numbers.

If a researcher fails to conform to restrictions 2 and 3, his or her calculated chi-square will not conform to the chi-square distribution table. The sampling distribution of the standardized score approximates the table only when qualifications 2 and 3 are met. If they are not met, the probability of obtaining the research results when the null hypothesis is true is *greater* than the table would indicate. Thus, although Table C.3 might indicate that the probability of the results is .05 or less, in actuality the probability may be greater than .05. Researchers who fail to take into account these restrictions are risking reporting results as significant when they are not significant. According to rule 3, if a 2×2 table is used and any expected frequency falls below 5, chi-square should not be calculated, because each cell represents 25 percent of the total number of expected frequencies in that case. Fortunately, when this is the case, there is an alternative statistic to apply to the data. It is called Fisher's exact test. While we will not go into how it is calculated, the student should be aware of its existence. Think of it as an alternative to the chi-square statistic that should be applied when one is working with a 2×2 table having any expected frequency under 5. Fisher's exact test can be applied *only* to a 2×2 table.[2]

The final qualification also refers only to 2×2 tables. A Yates correction for continuity consists of either adding or subtracting .5 to or from the *observed* frequencies in order to reduce the difference in size between the observed and the expected frequencies. Thus, if the expected frequency is larger than the observed, one adds .5 to the observed frequency. If the expected frequency is smaller than the

[2] For a complete discussion of Fisher's exact test, see Siegel (1956, pp. 96–104).

observed, one subtracts .5 from the observed frequency. This process reduces the size of the deviation between the observed and the expected value in each cell and thus has the effect of reducing the magnitude of the final chi-square value. The rationale for applying the Yates correction for continuity is similar to that for not applying chi-square when more than 20 percent of the expected values are less than 5.

By applying a Yates correction for continuity, the researcher is assured that the probability of the calculated chi-square value complies with the probability listed in the chi-square table. This process is illustrated for Table 9.3.

For Table 9.3 the application of a Yates correction for continuity reduces the chi-square value from 4.80 to 3.34. As with all 2×2 tables df $= 1$. Referring to Table C.3 we see that the minimum chi-square value to reject H_0 is 3.841. Thus we would have rejected H_0 when converting Table 9.3 to a chi-square score *without* applying the Yates correction

Table 9.3. Hospitalization During Previous 12 Months, by Sex

Sex	Hospitalization		Total
	Yes	No	
Male	2	18	20
Female	8	12	20
Total	10	30	$N = 40$

Calculation of Chi-Square for Table 9.3 Without Yates Correction for Continuity

O	E	$O-E$	$(O-E)^2$	$(O-E)^2/E$
2	5	−3	9	1.80
18	15	3	9	.60
8	5	3	9	1.80
12	15	−3	9	.60
				$\chi^2 = 4.80$

Calculation of Chi-Square for Table 9.3 With Yates Correction for Continuity

Corrected O	E	$O-E$	$(O-E)^2$	$(O-E)^2/E$
2.5	5	−2.5	6.25	1.25
17.5	15	2.5	6.25	.42
7.5	5	2.5	6.25	1.25
12.5	15	−2.5	6.25	.42
				$\chi^2 = 3.34$

for continuity, since 4.80 is *greater* than 3.841. On the other hand, when incorporating a Yates correction for continuity into the calculation we must accept H_0, since 3.34 is *less* than 3.841. The corrected chi-square value of 3.34 results in a more accurate estimation of the probability of obtaining Table 9.3 when the null hypothesis is true than the uncorrected value of 4.80. As in the present example, the application of the Yates correction for continuity can change the inference decision of whether to reject or accept the null hypothesis. It is therefore important to apply a Yates correction for continuity whenever one is working with a 2×2 table with any expected frequency between 5 and 10.

When evaluating research that used chi-square to analyze data, the reader should make sure that the author has conformed to the requirements regarding expected frequencies. The reader can do this by computing expected frequencies for the author's table(s). The author should let the reader know whether a Yates correction for continuity has been applied to the data.

Shortcut Formulas for the Calculation of Chi-Square

While the $\Sigma (O-E)^2/E$ formula can always be used to calculate a chi-square score, there are three alternative formulas that shorten the computations involved. Although the underlying logic of chi-square is not readily apparent in either of these formulas, they both have the advantage of simplifying the computational process. To illustrate their use, we will recalculate chi-square values for Table 9.1.

The following computational formula can be used *only* on a 2×2 table:

$$\chi^2 = \frac{N (AD - BC)^2}{(A+B) (C+D) (A+C) (B+D)} \tag{9.2}$$

where A = observed frequency in upper left cell
B = observed frequency in upper right cell
C = observed frequency in lower left cell
D = observed frequency in lower right cell
N = total number of cases

The cells and their marginal totals for Table 9.1 are shown below:

	A	B	Totals
	28	72	100 $(A+B)$
	C	D	
	32	18	50 $(C+D)$
	$(A+C)$ 60	$(B+D)$ 90	$N =$ 150

Applying this computational formula to these data we find

$$\chi^2 = \frac{150\,[(28)\,(18) - (72)\,(32)]^2}{(28+72)\,(32+18)\,(28+32)\,(72+18)}$$

$$= \frac{150\,(504-2304)^2}{(100)\,(50)\,(60)\,(90)}$$

$$= \frac{150\,(-1800)^2}{27,000,000}$$

$$= \frac{150\,(3,240,000)}{27,000,000} = \frac{486,000,000}{27,000,000} = 18.00$$

The second computational formula is not restricted to a 2×2 table. It can be applied to a table of any size.

$$\chi^2 = \Sigma\,\frac{O^2}{E} - N \qquad\qquad (9.3)$$

where O = observed frequency in a cell
E = expected frequency in a cell
N = total number of cases

Applying this formula to Table 9.1 entails the following computations:

Cell	O	O^2	E	O^2/E
A	28	784	40	19.6
B	72	5184	60	86.4
C	32	1024	20	51.2
D	18	324	30	10.8
				168.0

$$\Sigma\,\frac{O^2}{E} = 19.6 + 86.4 + 51.2 + 10.8$$

$$= 168$$

$$\Sigma\,\frac{O^2}{E} - N = 168 - 150$$

$$\chi^2 = 18.0$$

Finally, the formula shown below incorporates the Yates correction for continuity into the computational formula for a 2×2 table. It can be used whenever an *expected* frequency falls between 5 and 10 in a table of this size.

$$\chi^2 = \frac{N\,(|AD - BC| - N/2)^2}{(A+B)\,(C+D)\,(A+C)\,(B+D)} \qquad\qquad (9.4)$$

Applying formula 9.4 to Table 9.3 we obtain the following result:

$$\chi^2 = \frac{40\,[\,|(2)\,(12) - (18)\,(8)| - 40/2\,]^2}{(2+18)\,(8+12)\,(2+8)\,(18+12)}$$

$$= \frac{40\,[\,|24-144| - 20\,]^2}{(20)\,(20)\,(10)\,(30)} = \frac{40\,[\,|-120| - 20\,]^2}{120{,}000}$$

$$= \frac{40(100)^2}{120{,}000} = \frac{40(10{,}000)}{120{,}000} = \frac{400{,}000}{120{,}000} = 3.33$$

In Chapter 10 we consider several statistical tests especially suited to hypothesis testing with ordinal level data.

WORKING WITH AND INTERPRETING DATA

1. Refer again to question 2 at the end of Chapter 3. Construct a contingency table using the data on initiation of solid foods and La Leche League membership. Apply a chi-square test to your table and go through the seven-step hypothesis testing process.

2. Refer again to the Triplett article referenced in the questions at the end of Chapter 8. The author uses the chi-square test to evaluate differences between good and poor users of preventive health care services. In Table 2 on page 143 of the article she compares the two groups according to a variety of demographic variables. Using these data, complete the following:

   a. Calculate your own chi-square values for the data presented in Triplett's Table 2. In so doing, go through the seven-step hypothesis testing process.
   b. Evaluate Triplett's use of the chi-square statistic. Is chi-square appropriate in this instance? Has it been applied correctly? If not, explain why.
   c. Does Triplett apply a Yates correction for continuity to any of these data? If so, is her application justified?

3. Use the chi-square table (Appendix C, Table C.3) to make an inference decision for each of the following situations:

   a. $\chi^2 = 5.52$
      Level of Significance = .05
      2 × 2 table
   b. $\chi^2 = 15.21$
      Level of Significance = .01
      8 × 2 table

   c. $\chi^2 = 4.55$
     Level of Significance $= .05$
     2×3 table
   d. $\chi^2 = 9.66$
     Level of Significance $= .01$
     4×2 table

Hypothesis Testing with Ordinal Level Data

In this chapter we consider three statistical tests that are especially suited to ordinal level data: the median test, the Mann-Whitney U test, and the Wald-Wolfowitz runs test. All three are used for evaluating differences between two samples. However, the tests differ in the kinds of differences to which they are sensitive. Specifically, the median test judges whether two samples differ in terms of central tendency. The Mann-Whitney U test considers whether one sample has significantly higher ranks than another. The Wald-Wolfowitz runs test evaluates whether the two samples differ in *any* way (e.g., central tendency, variability). Each test is applied to the data according to the standard seven-step hypothesis testing format (see Chapter 9).

Median Test

Our students sometimes accuse us of unfair grading practices, complaining that one of us is a harder grader than the other. When this happens, we statistically evaluate the validity of the accusation. Data (grades given for one of our examinations) are presented in Table 10.1. These will be evaluated using the median test. The 29 students were randomly divided into two groups of 15 and 14 each for grading purposes.

The median test allows the researcher to determine the probability that two or more independent samples (not necessarily of the same size) have been drawn from a single population. If this is true, then the sample medians should be approximately equal. The test requires at least ordinal level data, so that a median can be computed. In the present example we have decided to treat examination scores as ordinal as opposed to interval data for two reasons. First, we are unwilling to assume that our measurement instrument (the examination) is sensitive enough to yield truly interval level data. Second, each distribution is negatively skewed, which makes the median a better indicator of central tendency than the mean in this case.

Testing a Null Hypothesis Using the Median Test

Step 1, H_1 : The median examination scores for the two groups differ. Since we are using the median to compare the two groups, we also can write H_1 in the following shortened form: $Md_1 \neq Md_2$. This is a nondirectional research hypothesis. Since we will be using the chi-square sampling distribution to determine the probability of the standardized score we calculate, we cannot state a directional research hypothesis.

Table 10.1. Examination Scores from Two Different Graders

Graded by Kviz (X_1)	Graded by Knafl (X_2)
33	39
62	61
73	70
77	73
79	74
82	77
82	77
85	82
91	85
91	88
91	89
94	91
100	94
100	100
100	

Step 2, H_0: There is no difference in the median examination scores for the two groups, or $Md_1 = Md_2$.

Step 3, Level of Significance: .05

Step 4, Sampling Distribution: We will convert the data to a chi-square standardized score and use the chi-square sampling distribution to determine the probability of obtaining that score when H_0 is true.

As we will see in step 6, in order to calculate the standardized score we must first cast the data into a 2 × 2 cross-classification table. Applying the formula for calculating degrees of freedom, we see that we will use the chi-square curve corresponding to 1 degree of freedom to determine the probability of the standardized score we calculate in this example.

$$df = (R - 1)(C - 1)$$
$$= (2 - 1)(2 - 1)$$
$$= 1$$

Step 5, Region of Rejection: Using Table C.3 we see that the minimum chi-square value needed to reject the null hypothesis at the .05 level of significance and 1 degree of freedom is 3.841. The region of rejection is depicted below.

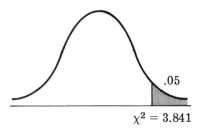

.05

$\chi^2 = 3.841$

Step 6, Standardized Score. We will convert these data into a chi-square standardized score. The difference between the median test and the chi-square test calculated in the previous chapter lies in the nature of the cross-classification table. The formula used for calculating the standardized score remains the same. When using the median test, the researcher divides the scores for each group according to whether or not they fall above or below the *combined* median of the groups.[1]

In order to do that, we have to determine the combined median of the two groups, count the number of scores in each group that fall above the combined median and the number of scores that fall below the combined median, and enter the resultant frequencies in a 2×2 table. If H_0 is true, we would expect approximately half of each instructor's scores to fall *above* the combined median and approximately half to fall *below* the combined median. The calculations entailed in these three steps are shown in Table 10.2. The cross-classification shown in step 3 of Table 10.2 can now be converted into a standardized chi-square score using the computational formula of $\chi^2 = \Sigma(O^2/E) - N$ presented in the previous chapter. The calculation of the chi-square score is summarized in Table 10.3. Note that a Yates correction for continuity has been incorporated into these calculations, since we have expected frequencies falling between 5 and 10. The resultant chi-square score is .04.

Step 7, Inference Decision: Comparing the calculated standardized score of .04 with the minimum chi-square score of 3.841 needed to reject the null hypothesis, we see that our chi-square value is smaller than 3.841 and thus accept the null hypothesis. In so doing we recognize that we are risking a type II error. Results of a median test should be reported in the same format as used for the chi-square test in Chapter 9. Whenever a Yates correction for continuity is applied to the data, this should be communicated to the reader in a footnote.

The Mann-Whitney U Test

Like the median test, the Mann-Whitney U test lets us determine the probability that two independent samples have been drawn from the same population. Specifically, this test evaluates whether the summed ranks of one group are significantly higher than those of the other group (see discussion under step 6 of this section).

---

[1] If a number of scores fall exactly at the median, the researcher can decide to divide scores into either (1) those falling at or above and those falling below the combined median *or* (2) those falling at or below and those falling above the combined median.

Table 10.2. Calculating the Combined Median for the Two Groups and Casting the Data into a 2×2 Table

Step 1: Calculate the combined median.

Score	f	cf	
33	1	1	$Md = L + \left(\dfrac{\dfrac{N}{2} - cf}{f} \cdot i \right)$
39	1	2	
61	1	3	$= 81.5 \left(\dfrac{14.5 - 12}{3} \cdot 1 \right)$
62	1	4	
70	1	5	$= 81.5 + \left(\dfrac{2.5}{3} \right)$
73	2	7	
74	1	8	$= 81.5 + .83$
77	3	11	
79	1	12	
82	3	15 ← Median	$= 82.33$
85	2	17 interval	
88	1	18	
89	1	19	
91	4	23	
94	2	25	
100	4	29	

Step 2: Determine the number of scores in each group that fall above and the number that fall below the combined median of 82.33.

Graded by Kviz

33	
62	
73	Below combined
77	median
79	
82	
82	
85	
91	Above combined
91	median
91	
94	
100	
100	
100	

Graded by Knafl

39	
61	
70	Below combined
73	median
74	
77	
77	
82	
85	
88	
89	Above combined
91	median
94	
100	

Step 3: Construct a cross-classification table.

	Kviz's scores	Knafl's scores	Total
Above median	8	6	14
Below median	7	8	15
Total	15	14	$N = 29$

Table 10.3. Calculation of Chi-Square Score

Cell	O (observed frequency)	CO (corrected observed frequency)	E (expected frequency)	$(CO)^2$	$(CO)^2/E$
A	8	7.5	7.24	56.25	7.77
B	6	6.5	6.76	42.25	6.25
C	7	7.5	7.76	56.25	7.25
D	8	7.5	7.24	56.25	7.77

$$\Sigma(CO)^2/E = 29.04$$

$$\chi^2 = \Sigma\frac{(CO)^2}{E} - N$$

$$= 29.04 - 29$$

$$= .04$$

For example, Knafl is currently involved in designing a study to determine if certain "experimental" nursing procedures will reduce preoperative anxiety in children. Those involved in the study anticipate comparing two groups of children: those receiving the "special care" (the experimental group), and those receiving no special attention (the control group). It is being hypothesized that the control group will have higher overall anxiety than the experimental.

Anxiety is difficult to measure, and whatever tool is devised or adopted, it is likely to be one that measures the data at the ordinal level. Anxiety scores will indicate whether a subject has more or less anxiety in comparison with others studied. Thus, anxiety scores will be treated as ordinal level data. Table 10.4 shows some hypothetical anxiety scores of the kind that might be found in the proposed study.

Table 10.4. Preoperative Anxiety Scores for Experimental and Control Groups

Experimental	Control
62	73
63	75
69	77
71	78
74	81
76	85
80	88
84	89
87	90
92	95
$N_1 = 10$	$N_2 = 10$

Testing a Null Hypothesis Using the Mann-Whitney U Test

Step 1, H_1 : Members of the control group will have anxiety scores that rank significantly higher than those of the experimental group. A directional research hypothesis is stated in this instance, since the purpose of the research is to evaluate a nursing intervention intended to reduce preoperative anxiety in children.

Step 2, H_0 : There will be no difference in rank between the anxiety scores of experimental and control group subjects.

Step 3, Level of Significance: .05.

Step 4, Sampling Distribution: In step 6 these data will be converted into a standardized score called a U score. The sampling distribution of U scores is summarized in Table C.4 (Appendix C). If this table is used, N_2, the size of the larger of the two samples, must be between 9 and 20. If N_2 is less than 9, we would use a slightly different table to find the probability of our standardized score. If N_2 is larger than 20, it is possible to convert the data to a z score and use the normal probability table to interpret our results.[2] In the present example the two groups are of equal size, but this is not always the case.

Table C.4 is set up and interpreted somewhat differently from the sampling distributions encountered thus far. The most important difference is that the values in the body of the table are the *maximum* score we can calculate and still be able to reject H_0. In other words, we can reject H_0 if we calculate a U score equal to or *less* than the critical value listed in the table. All other sampling distributions we have discussed depict either probabilities or *minimum* standardized scores needed to reject H_0 in the body of the table.

Step 5, Region of Rejection: We will use subtable C.4c, since our hypothesis is directional and the level of significance is .05. In order to find the maximum U score we can calculate and still be able to reject H_0, we find the value corresponding to the intersection of the N_2 row that runs across the top of Table C.4c and the N_1 column that runs down the left side. For the example we have been working with, we look for the intersection of $N_1 = 10$ and $N_2 = 10$. This value is 27. Thus, if we calculate a U score of 27 or *smaller*, we will reject H_0 at the .05 level of significance.

Step 6, Standardized Score: In applying the Mann-Whitney U test, we determine if the sum of the ranks assigned to one

---

[2] For a complete discussion of calculating a U test for different sample sizes see Siegel (1956, pp. 116–126).

group is significantly greater than the sum of the ranks assigned to the other group. For the present example, we are predicting that the sum of the ranks of the control group will be greater than the sum of the ranks of the experimental group. The first step in converting the raw data (the anxiety scores) into a standardized U score is to put together the scores of both groups and give each score a rank, assigning the rank of 1 to the lowest score, 2 to the next lowest score, and so on (see Table 10.5). In distributions where there are tied scores these are assigned the average of the tied ranks. Thus, in the current examples, if the three lowest scores had been 62, 62, and 69 instead of 62, 63, and 69, both scores of 62 would have received a rank of 1.5 (the average of ranks 1 and 2). The score of 69 would have been assigned a rank of 3 as in the current example. Once all 20 scores have been ranked, the sum of the ranks for each group is found. It is the value of the summed ranks that is used in the calculation of

Table 10.5. Combined Ranking and Summed Ranks for Experimental and Control Groups

Rank	Score	Rank	Score
1	62	11	80
2	63	12	81
3	69	13	84
4	71	14	85
5	73	15	87
6	74	16	88
7	75	17	89
8	76	18	90
9	77	19	92
10	78	20	95

Experimental (N_1)		Control (N_1)	
Score	Rank	Score	Rank
62	1	73	5
63	2	75	7
69	3	77	9
71	4	78	10
74	6	81	12
76	8	85	14
80	11	88	16
84	13	89	17
87	15	90	18
92	19	95	20
	$R_1 = 82$		$R_2 = 128$

a U score. Table 10.5 shows the combined ranking of all 20 scores and the summed ranks for the experimental and control groups.

The summed ranks are converted to a standardized U score through one or the other of the following formulas:

$$U = N_1 N_2 + \frac{N_1 (N_1 + 1)}{2} - R_1 \qquad (10.1)$$

or

$$U = N_1 N_2 + \frac{N_2 (N_2 + 1)}{2} - R_2 \qquad (10.2)$$

where N_1 = number of subjects in the smaller of the two samples
N_2 = number of subjects in the larger of the two samples
R_1 = sum of ranks assigned to sample N_1
R_2 = sum of ranks assigned to sample N_2

Formulas 10.1 and 10.2 yield different U values. In order for Table C.4 to reflect accurately the probability of obtaining the observed results when H_0 is true, we must use the *smaller* value as U; the larger value is called U' (U prime). We find U by substituting appropriate values in *both* formulas and then using the *smaller* value when looking up the probability of the result in Table C.4. Table 10.6 shows the calculation of U using both formulas. In this case formula 10.2 yields the smaller value. Therefore $U = 27$ and $U' = 73$.

We can always differentiate between U and U' by substituting appropriate values in both formulas. An easier method is to calculate the standardized score by using *either* formula 10.1 or 10.2 and then solve the following formula for U' to see if U or U' has been calculated:

$$U = N_1 N_2 - U' \qquad (10.3)$$

In formula 10.1 we calculated a U value of 73. Substituting this value in formula 10.3 and solving for U' we find

$U' = (10) (10) - 73$

$U' = 100 - 73$

$U' = 27$

Since 27 is smaller than 73, we now know that 27 is the U score and 73 is U'. We use the value of 27 when making an inference decision.

Table 10.6. Calculation of U Score

1. *Calculation using formula 10.1*

$$U = N_1 N_2 + \frac{N_1 (N_1 + 1)}{2} - R_1$$

$$= (10)(10) + \frac{10(11)}{2} - 82$$

$$= 100 + 55 - 82$$

$$= 73$$

2. *Calculation using formula 10.2*

$$U = N_1 N_2 + \frac{N_2 (N_2 + 1)}{2} - R_2$$

$$= (10)(10) + \frac{10(11)}{2} - 128$$

$$= 100 + 55 - 128$$

$$= 27$$

3. *Therefore $U = 27$ and $U' = 73$*

Step 7, Inference Decision: In step 5 we established that if we calculated a U score of 27 or less we reject H_0. Since $U = 27$, we reject H_0 in favor of the research hypothesis. In rejecting H_0 we are risking a type I error.

Wald-Wolfowitz Runs Test

In contrast to the median test, which is sensitive to differences in central tendency, and the Mann-Whitney U test, which focuses on differences in rank, the Wald-Wolfowitz runs test indicates whether two independent samples have been drawn from populations that differ in *any* way. We will apply the Wald-Wolfowitz runs test to the same data we used for the Mann-Whitney U test and will then compare the results of the two tests.

Testing a Null Hypothesis Using the Wald-Wolfowitz Runs Test

Step 1, H_1 : There is a significant difference between the anxiety scores of experimental and control group subjects. Since the Wald-Wolfowitz runs test is a general test of difference between groups, we state a nondirectional research hypothesis.

Step 2, H_0: There is no difference between anxiety scores of subjects in the experimental and the control group.

Step 3, Level of Significance: .05.

Step 4, Sampling Distribution: In step 6 we will be calculating the number of "runs" in the data presented in Table 10.4. This number is called an *r value*. Table C.5 gives the *r* values needed to reject H_0 for various sample sizes. Note that Table C.5 accommodates sample groups of between 2 and 20 only. When *either* group is larger than 20, this table cannot be used to determine the probability of the results if H_0 is true. With samples larger than 20 it is possible to convert the *r* value to a *z* score and use the normal probability table to interpret the data.[3] As with the sampling distribution for the Mann-Whitney *U* test, we will reject H_0 if our calculated *r* value is equal to or *smaller* than the critical value listed in the body of Table C.5.

Step 5, Region of Rejection: In order to find the maximum *r* value at which we can still reject H_0, we find the value corresponding to the intersection of the row and column representing the size of each group. In this case we are interested in the $N_1 = 10$ row and $N_2 = 10$ column. This value is 6. Thus, if we calculate an *r* value of 6 or less, we will reject H_0.

Step 6, Standardized Score: To calculate an *r* value we rank together the scores of each group, keeping track of whether each ranked score belongs to an experimental or a control subject. We then count the number of *runs*, or clusters of subjects, from each group. This process is shown in Table 10.7. Looking at Table 10.7, you can see that a maximum clustering of subjects in each group would yield two runs. This would happen if, for example, the experimental subjects fell into ranks 1–10 and the control subjects fell into ranks 11–20. This is the smallest *r* value possible. On the other hand the maximum *r* value possible is 20 and represents a minimum clustering of subjects from each group. This would occur if experimental subjects fell into all the even-numbered ranks and control subjects fell into the odd-numbered ranks or vice versa. In the present example the *r* value of 14 indicates that we are between these two extremes.

Step 7, Inference Decision: In step 5 we established that if we had 6 or fewer runs in the data, we would reject H_0. Since we had 14 runs, we accept H_0. In making this decision we are risking a type II error.

[3] For a complete discussion of this see Siegel (1956, pp. 140–143).

Table 10.7. Combined Ranking of Experimental (E) and Control (C) Subjects and Calculation of Total Number of Runs

Rank	Score	Group	
1	62	E	
2	63	E	Run 1
3	69	E	
4	71	E	
5	73	C	Run 2
6	74	E	Run 3
7	75	C	Run 4
8	76	E	Run 5
9	77	C	Run 6
10	78	C	
11	80	E	Run 7
12	81	C	Run 8
13	84	E	Run 9
14	85	C	Run 10
15	87	E	Run 11
16	88	C	
17	89	C	Run 12
18	90	C	
19	92	E	Run 13
20	95	C	Run 14

Comparison of Mann-Whitney U Test and Wald-Wolfowitz Runs Test

This decision perhaps strikes the reader as somewhat curious, since when using the Mann-Whitney U test we were able to reject H_0 for the same set of data. The difference in inference decision arises because the Mann-Whitney U test is a more *powerful* test than the Wald-Wolfowitz runs test. The power of any test has to do with the probability of rejecting the null hypothesis when it is false. The more likely it is that a specific statistical test will reject a *false* null hypothesis, the more powerful that particular test. Statisticians have estimated the comparative power of many statistical tests. By taking into account the exact rankings of the observations, the Mann-Whitney U test utilizes more information than the Wald-Wolfowitz runs tests, and this is the source of its greater power. The reader must also keep in mind that the two tests are sensitive to different kinds of differences between samples. The Mann-Whitney U test is sensitive to differences in ranking. Using it, the investigator can determine if one sample ranks significantly higher than another. The Wald-Wolfowitz runs test, on the other hand, tests whether the *populations* that the samples represent differ in any way. The purpose of the proposed study is to determine if the experimental group shows less anxiety than the control group. Therefore it is appropriate to apply the Mann-Whitney U test to the data, since we are interested in the specific kind of difference this test measures.

WORKING WITH AND INTERPRETING DATA

1. In the questions at the end of Chapter 9 you were asked to apply a chi-square test to the data on La Leche League membership and the initiation of solid foods first presented in the problem section at the end of Chapter 3. Now apply a median test to the data, going through the entire hypothesis testing process. Use the class intervals you established previously and the interpolation formula to calculate a median for these data. Compare the results of the two tests. Do you think that the chi-square or the median test is more appropriate in this instance?

2. The following hypothetical data represent satisfaction scores for two samples of staff nurses, one a group of nurses working in a hospital that has primary care nursing and the other a group working in a hospital that has team nursing.

Team Care Scores	Primary Care Scores
28	99
54	94
75	65
68	90
83	98
36	90
60	75
61	81
49	88
78	84
85	
71	
67	

a. Use a Mann-Whitney U test to test the following research hypothesis: The satisfaction scores of nurses working in a primary care setting will rank significantly higher than the scores of those working in a team care setting.

b. Apply a Wald-Wolfowitz runs test to these same data. What is the research hypothesis being tested in this case?

c. Compare the results of these two tests and comment on the appropriateness of each.

3. The following articles contain examples of hypothesis testing with ordinal level data. For each example, describe and interpret the author's findings and evaluate the author's use of the particular statistical value.

Davis, Betty G. Clinical expertise as a function of educational preparation. *Nursing Research* 21:530, 1972.

Eggland, Ellen T. Locus of control and children with cerebral palsy. *Nursing Research* 22:329, 1973.

Mulcahy, Rae A., and Janz, N. Effectiveness of raising pain perception threshold in males and females using a psychoprophylactic childbirth technique during induced pain. *Nursing Research* 22:423, 1973.

Hypothesis Testing with Interval Level Data

In the previous two chapters we have considered various techniques of evaluating observed differences between sample groups measured at the nominal and ordinal levels. In this chapter we direct our attention to statistical tests appropriate for interval level data. Specifically, we will consider techniques for comparing the means of two sample groups. These techniques make it possible to determine the probability that the observed differences between the means of two or more random samples reflect corresponding differences in the populations from which they were selected. While focusing on ways to compare the means of two samples, we also introduce a method of comparing sample means of more than two groups. Techniques for comparing *two* sample means are called *difference-between-means tests* or often, to sound less cumbersome, *t tests*. The comparison of means from *three* or more groups is accomplished through an analysis of variance, known simply as *ANOVA*.

Differences Between Means: An Example and Overview

A difference-between-means test is commonly used when the researcher has interval data and wants to determine if two groups have significantly different means. As in the statistical tests already discussed, the difference is evaluated by converting raw data into a standardized score and using a sampling distribution to find the probability of obtaining the calculated score when the null hypothesis is true.

For example, Gorman (1978) undertook a study of the comparative advantages and disadvantages of the CircOlectric bed and the logrolling technique for turning postoperative scoliosis patients. The data showing the numbers of hours slept the first postoperative day for subjects in each group is shown in Table 11.1.

As Table 11.1 shows, the means for these two groups are different. By converting this observed difference of 2.65 hours (9.30—6.65) into a standardized score, we will be able to determine the probability that the observed differences between the samples of patients treated with the CircOlectric bed and logrolled patients also would hold for the larger populations from which they were randomly drawn.

Like all the tests we have discussed so far, difference-between-means tests are based on specific assumptions about the nature of the data. As usual, we must conform to the requirement of random sampling. In addition, the application of a difference-between-means test requires interval level data. Thus, if a researcher wants to evaluate differences

Table 11.1. Number of Hours Slept First Postoperative Day for Patients in CircOlectric Bed and for Logrolled Patients

X_1 Logrolled (N = 10)	X_2 CircOlectric (N = 10)
11	12
6	3
11	2
12	2
9	4
15	2
9	10
7	11.5
3	8
10	12
$\Sigma X_1 = 93$	$\Sigma X_2 = 66.5$
$\overline{X}_1 = 9.30$	$\overline{X}_2 = 6.65$

between groups but has nominal or ordinal level data, he or she would have to choose from among the techniques described in the previous two chapters.

Unlike the hypothesis testing techniques discussed thus far, difference-between-means tests are based on the assumption that the variable in question is normally distributed in the populations and that the population variances are approximately equal.[1] The data should conform to all these requirements before the researcher would use a difference-between-means test.

Having met these requirements, the researcher still faces several decisions regarding the use of the test. The specific procedures for calculating and interpreting a difference-between-means test will vary somewhat depending on the following:

1. Whether the combined sample size is large (100 or greater) or small
2. Whether each group contains the same number of subjects
3. Whether sample groups are *independent* of one another or are *related* (the same sample measured at two different times)

[1] Statistical tests, in general, can be divided into two broad groups, those that make certain assumptions about the nature of the population from which the data were drawn and those that do not make such assumptions. The former are called *parametric* statistical tests; the latter are called *nonparametric* statistical tests. Unlike the statistical tests presented in Chapters 9 and 10, those discussed in the present chapter are parametric statistical tests. For a fuller discussion of the differences between parametric and nonparametric statistical tests, see Siegel (1956, pp. 30–34).

Combined sample size is the main determinant of whether one uses the normal probability sampling distribution or the t-sampling distribution to interpret results.[2] We will discuss this consideration in detail under step 4 of the hypothesis testing process. Points 2 and 3 introduce slight differences into the calculations of the standardized score. These will be presented under step 6.

It should be emphasized that in spite of these differences all difference-between-means tests discussed in this chapter share a common underlying logic: Computation of a standardized score based on the differences between the means of *two* sample groups to determine the probability that the observed sample differences would also hold true for the populations from which the samples were drawn.

Testing a Null Hypothesis Using a Difference-Between-Means Test

In this section we will use the data from the logrolling-vs.-CircOlectric bed study to demonstrate testing a hypothesis using a difference-between-means test.

Step 1, H_1: There is a difference between patients treated by logrolling and those treated by the CircOlectric bed in number hours slept during the first postoperative day. Since we are using the means to compare the two groups, we can present H_1 in the following, summarized form: $\overline{X}_1 \neq \overline{X}_2$. This is a *nondirectional* research hypothesis. While it is possible to state a directional hypothesis when using a difference-between-means test, the researcher did not feel justified in doing so in this case. Thus, although Gorman expected to find some differences between logrolled patients and those treated with the CircOlectric bed, she was not willing to make specific predictions about the nature of those differences.

Step 2, H_0: There is no difference between patients treated by logrolling and those treated by the CircOlectric bed in number of hours slept during the first postoperative day, or $\overline{X}_1 = \overline{X}_2$.

Step 3, Level of Significance: .05.

Step 4, Sampling Distribution: The sampling distribution we will use to interpret our results depends on the size of the *combined* sample (the total number of subjects in both groups). When the combined sample size is sufficiently large, 100 or more cases, the normal probability curve (Table C.2) is used to find the probability of the calculated standardized score if H_0 is true. When the combined sample size is under

---

[2] For a more complete discussion of issues involved in this decision, see Loether and McTavish (1974b, pp. 95–97).

100, the *t* distribution is used to find the probability of the standardized score. This is because, when the sample is large, the sampling distribution of standardized difference-between-means scores approximates a normal probability distribution. When the combined sample size is smaller than 100, the sampling distribution of standardized scores no longer conforms to the normal probability curve. Rather, it approximates the *t* distribution, which is summarized in Table C.6 of Appendix C.

Like the chi-square distribution, the *t* distribution is a family of curves. Which curve the researcher uses to find the probability of a particular standardized score depends on the size of the combined sample. In Table C.6 sample size is taken into account under the degrees of freedom (df) column. The number of degrees of freedom for a difference-between-means test based on data from *independent* random samples, as in the present example, equals the combined sample size minus 2. When data from *related* samples are analyzed, degrees of freedom equals the number of subjects minus 1.[3] We will apply these principles in step 5 when we specify the region of rejection.

Because in the present example the combined sample size is less than 100, we will use the *t* distribution to interpret our results. We will call the standardized score a *t* score. When the normal probability curve is used to interpret the standardized score, the score is called a *z score*. Whether the resultant standardized value is called a *z* score or a *t* score, the calculations and interpretation of results remain the same. In spite of this distinction, researchers frequently use the term *t test* generically to refer to any difference-between-means test regardless of the sampling distribution being used to interpret the results.

Step 5, Region of Rejection: Since we have stated a nondirectional research hypothesis and our level of significance is .05, the region of rejection is equally divided between the negative and the positive tails of the appropriate *t* curve.

In order to determine the minimum *t* value needed to reject the null hypothesis in this case, the reader must know how to use Table C.6, which sets forth the *t* distribution. Each row in Table C.6 summarizes a separate *t* curve. Degrees of freedom determines with which row of the *t* table the researcher is concerned. For this example, degrees of freedom equals 18.

$$df = N - 2$$
$$= 20 - 2$$
$$= 18$$

---

[3] For a general discussion of the concept of degrees of freedom as it relates to the *t* distribution, the student is referred to Loether and McTavish (1974b, pp. 97–98).

Thus, we are interested in the eighteenth row of the t table.

The table also takes into account whether the researcher has stated a directional or a nondirectional research hypothesis. The two rows of probability levels (beginning with .10 for one-tailed and .20 for two-tailed tests) are lined up over columns of numbers that correspond to the minimum standardized score (t value) needed to reject the null hypothesis at a certain level of significance for a given degree of freedom. For this example we find the value that corresponds to the intersection of 18 degrees of freedom and a level of significance of .05 for a two-tailed research hypothesis. The value we find is ± 2.101, which is the minimum t value needed to reject the null hypothesis. Note that if the researcher had stated a directional (one-tailed) hypothesis, a t value of 1.734 would have been sufficient to reject the null hypothesis. This is consistent with the fact that it is always easier to reject the null hypothesis when one has stated a directional as opposed to a nondirectional research hypothesis.

It is important to remember that, when stating a directional hypothesis, the researcher is predicting *either* a positive or a negative standardized score. This means that if a positive score is predicted, but a negative score is calculated, the researcher *cannot* reject the null hypothesis, no matter how large the calculated standardized score is. Since research hypotheses are formulated prior to the collection of data, this is not an unheard-of occurrence. For the example we are using, we can picture the region of rejection in the following way:

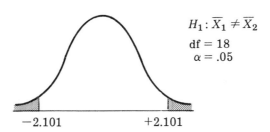

$H_1 : \overline{X}_1 \neq \overline{X}_2$
df = 18
$\alpha = .05$

−2.101   +2.101

If we were working with a large sample (combined sample size of 100 or more), we would use the normal probability curve to interpret the standardized score. Because the normal curve is a single distribution and not a family of curves like the t distribution, we need not concern ourselves with degrees of freedom. We simply use the normal probability curve to find the probability of the standardized score we have calculated. At the .05 level of significance the probability has to be .05 or less for a one-tailed test and .025 or less for a two-tailed test before we can reject the null hypothesis. This situation is depicted as follows:

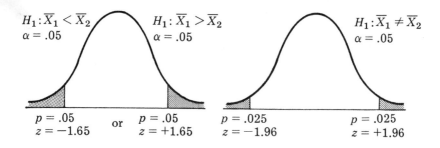

$H_1: \overline{X}_1 < \overline{X}_2$
$\alpha = .05$

$H_1: \overline{X}_1 > \overline{X}_2$
$\alpha = .05$

$H_1: \overline{X}_1 \neq \overline{X}_2$
$\alpha = .05$

$p = .05$ or $p = .05$ $p = .025$ $p = .025$
$z = -1.65$ $z = +1.65$ $z = -1.96$ $z = +1.96$

We can now turn our attention to converting the raw data into a standardized score.

Step 6, Standardized Score: As was noted at the outset of this chapter, certain differences exist in the standardization procedure depending on whether the two samples are the same size and whether they are independent or related. Since we are working with two independent samples of the same size in our current example, we will discuss first the standardization formula used for samples of the same size. Later we will show how this formula varies when one is working with samples of unequal size or related samples.

The standardization of the difference between the means of the CircOlectric and logrolling treatments is accomplished by applying the following formula to the data:

$$t = \frac{\overline{X}_1 - \overline{X}_2}{\sigma_{diff}} \qquad (11.1)$$

where $\overline{X}_1$ = mean of the first group
       $\overline{X}_2$ = mean of the second group
       σ_{diff} = standard deviation of the sampling distribution
                 of differences between means, known as the
                 standard error of the difference

The formula entails dividing the difference between the two sample means by a special kind of standard deviation, called the *standard error of the difference*.

The standard error of the difference is the name for the standard deviation of a sampling distribution made up of all possible difference-between-means scores. You will never be called upon to generate such a sampling distribution, but a basic understanding of its nature is essential for understanding the standardization formula for the difference-between-means test.

In order to grasp this concept, imagine a situation in which a researcher repeatedly draws two random samples of a given size from a single population. Under this condition, since the samples represent the same population, no difference is expected between their means. In other words, this is the expected outcome when the null hypothesis is true.

The researcher computes a mean for each sample and then sub-tracts the mean of the first sample from the mean of the second sample, thereby generating a difference score. If the researcher continues this process until all possible pairs of samples have been drawn and difference of means scores calculated, it would then be possible to generate a sampling distribution of the difference-between-means scores. Such a distribution is depicted below.

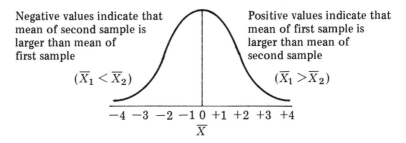

Negative values indicate that mean of second sample is larger than mean of first sample

$(\overline{X}_1 < \overline{X}_2)$

Positive values indicate that mean of first sample is larger than mean of second sample

$(\overline{X}_1 > \overline{X}_2)$

$$-4 \ -3 \ -2 \ -1 \ 0 \ +1 \ +2 \ +3 \ +4$$
$$\overline{X}$$

Note that such a sampling distribution approximates a normal curve and its mean would be zero. Thus, over a large number of cases, as in our hypothetical example, the most typical or "average" difference score would be zero. As the illustration shows, small difference scores are more probable and thus fall near the center of the curve. The larger difference scores, be-cause they are less probable, fall into the upper or lower tails of the curve. A positive difference score is obtained when the mean of the first sample is larger than the mean of the second sample; a negative difference score is generated when the mean of the first sample is less than the mean of the second sample.

As with any distribution, a standard deviation can be cal-culated for this one. In this instance the resulting standard deviation is called the *standard error of the difference* and is symbolized σ_{diff}. It is this standard error of the difference that goes into the denominator of the formula for calculating a t score. The reader should recognize a similarity between the formula for a t score and that for a z score presented in Chapter 7. In both cases we are dividing a deviation score $(X - \overline{X}$ or $\overline{X}_1 - \overline{X}_2)$ by a standard deviation (σ or σ_{diff}).

We estimate this standard error of the difference on the basis of something called the *standard error.* The standard error, which is also a special kind of standard deviation, is es-timated on the basis of the standard deviation of the two samples. The standard error, symbolized $\sigma_{\overline{X}}$, is a standard deviation for a sampling distribution of means. Like the sampling distribution of difference scores on which the stan-dard error of the difference is based, the sampling distribution of means is something you will never be called upon to gener-ate. This is because it is possible to estimate the standard error on the basis of the standard deviation of each of the two samples. At the same time you should have a basic under-standing of the concept of standard error.

Imagine a situation in which a researcher draws all possible samples of a given size from a population. For each such sample the mean value for some variable of interest is calculated. These mean values can then be used to generate a sampling distribution of means. As in the case of the sampling distribution of difference scores, the sampling distribution of means will approximate a normal curve, but its mean will equal the mean of the population from which the samples were drawn.[4] Sample means that deviate greatly from the population mean are comparatively improbable and will thus be found in the tails of the sampling distribution.

In sum, to calculate a standardized t value the researcher must make an estimate of the standard error of the difference. He or she does this by making an estimate of the standard error on the basis of the standard deviation of each of the two samples.

In actual practice the researcher begins by calculating the mean and standard deviation for each sample, using the familiar formulas repeated below.

$$\bar{X} = \frac{\Sigma fX}{N} \tag{11.2}$$

$$\sigma = \sqrt{\frac{\Sigma fX^2}{N} - \bar{X}^2} \tag{11.3}[5]$$

Having made these calculations it is possible to estimate both the standard error and the standard error of the difference by using the following formulas.

$$\sigma_{\bar{X}} = \frac{\sigma}{\sqrt{N}} \tag{11.4}$$

$$\sigma_{diff} = \sqrt{\sigma_{\bar{X}_1}^2 + \sigma_{\bar{X}_2}^2} \tag{11.5}$$

The standard error is calculated for each sample by dividing the standard deviation of that sample by the square root of

---

[4] This is known as the *central limit theorem*. It states that, if repeated random samples of size N are drawn from a normally distributed population with mean μ and standard deviation σ, the means of such samples will be normally distributed, with the mean equaling μ and standard error equaling $\sigma/\sqrt{N}$. For a complete discussion of the central limit theorem, see Loether and McTavish (1974b, pp. 93–95).

[5] Often in statistics a distinction is made between statistics based on data from a sample and those based on data from a population. This is done by using Greek letters such as "σ" to designate statistics based on population data and Roman letters such as "s" to designate statistics based on sample data. However, for the sake of clarity and simplicity we have chosen not to make this distinction and have used the same symbol for a given statistic throughout the text.

the sample size. The standard error of the difference is the square root of the sum of the squared standard error estimates. The reader now has all the information necessary to compute the denominator of the formula for the t value (formula 11.1). The numerator of the formula entails simply subtracting the mean of the second group from the mean of the first group. The actual calculation of a t value for the present example is presented in Table 11.2. Having converted the raw data to a standardized score of 1.58, we can now make an inference decision regarding the null hypothesis.

Step 7, Inference Decision: Comparing our calculated standardized score of 1.58 with the minimum t score of 2.101 needed to reject the null hypothesis, we see that our t score is smaller than 2.101, and therefore accept the null hypothesis. Thus we cannot generalize our sample results to the populations from which the samples were drawn. In making this inference decision, we recognize that we are risking a type II error.

Our testing of the example used throughout this discussion is summarized below:

1. H_1 : There is a difference between the CircOlectric bed and logrolling treatment in the average number of hours patients spend sleeping the first postoperative day ($\overline{X}_1 \neq \overline{X}_2$).
2. H_0 : There is no difference between the CircOlectric bed and logrolling treatment in the average number of hours patients spend sleeping the first postoperative day ($\overline{X}_1 = \overline{X}_2$).
3. Level of significance: .05.
4. Sampling distribution: The t distribution with 18 degrees of freedom will be used to interpret the standardized score, since the combined sample size is under 100.
5. Region of rejection:

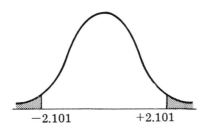

$-2.101 \qquad +2.101$

Table 11.2. Steps in Calculating a t Value

Step 1: Calculate $\overline{X}_1$ and $\overline{X}_2$.

$$\overline{X} = \frac{\Sigma fX}{N}$$

$$\overline{X}_1 = \frac{93}{10} \qquad\qquad\qquad \overline{X}_2 = \frac{66.5}{10}$$

$$= 9.30 \qquad\qquad\qquad\qquad = 6.65$$

Step 2: Calculate the standard deviation for each sample.

$$\sigma = \sqrt{\frac{\Sigma fX^2}{N} - \overline{X}^2}$$

$$\sigma_1 = \sqrt{\frac{967}{10} - 86.49} \qquad\qquad \sigma_2 = \sqrt{\frac{621.25}{10} - 44.22}$$

$$= \sqrt{96.70 - 86.49} \qquad\qquad\qquad = \sqrt{62.12 - 44.22}$$

$$= \sqrt{10.21} \qquad\qquad\qquad\qquad = \sqrt{17.90}$$

$$= \quad 3.20 \qquad\qquad\qquad\qquad = \quad 4.23$$

Step 3: Calculate the standard error for each sample.

$$\sigma_{\overline{X}} = \frac{\sigma}{\sqrt{N}}$$

$$\sigma_{\overline{X}_1} = \frac{3.20}{\sqrt{10}} \qquad\qquad\qquad \sigma_{\overline{X}_2} = \frac{4.23}{\sqrt{10}}$$

$$= \frac{3.20}{3.16} \qquad\qquad\qquad\qquad = \frac{4.23}{3.16}$$

$$= 1.01 \qquad\qquad\qquad\qquad = 1.34$$

Step 4: Calculate the standard error of the difference.

$$\sigma_{\text{diff}} = \sqrt{\sigma_{\overline{X}_1}{}^2 + \sigma_{\overline{X}_2}{}^2}$$

$$\sigma_{\text{diff}} = \sqrt{1.01^2 + 1.34^2}$$

$$= \sqrt{1.02 + 1.80}$$

$$= \sqrt{2.82}$$

$$= \quad 1.68$$

Step 5: Calculate standardized score.

$$t = \frac{\overline{X}_1 - \overline{X}_2}{\sigma_{\text{diff}}}$$

$$t = \frac{9.30 - 6.65}{1.68}$$

$$= 1.58$$

6. Standardized score:

$$t = \frac{\overline{X}_1 - \overline{X}_2}{\sqrt{\sigma_{\overline{X}_1}^2 + \sigma_{\overline{X}_2}^2}}$$

$$= 1.58$$

7. Inference decision: Accept H_0.

In discussing these findings the author might say something like the following:

The data yielded a t value of 1.58, which is not significant at the .05 level when a two-tailed test is used. This finding indicates that there is no significant difference in the number of hours slept the first post-operative day for the two groups.

Having summarized the findings, the researcher would be free to speculate in the "Discussion" section of the report as to why no difference exists between groups, e.g., discuss problems of research design, validity, and reliability of measurements as well as psychological and physiological factors.

Variations on the Calculation of the Standardized Score

The comparison of samples of unequal size or related samples requires certain adjustments in the formula for calculating the standardized score. When calculating a t value for samples of unequal size, the following formula should be used to estimate σ_{diff}:

$$\sigma_{diff} = \sqrt{\left(\frac{N_1 \sigma_1^2 + N_2 \sigma_2^2}{N_1 + N_2 - 2} \right) \left(\frac{1}{N_1} + \frac{1}{N_2} \right)} \qquad (11.6)$$

where σ_1 = standard deviation of the first sample

σ_2 = standard deviation of the second sample

N_1 = total number in first sample

N_2 = total number in second sample

What the above formula does is to weight the relative contribution of each sample to the estimate of the standard error of the difference, so that the larger sample contributes more to the final value than the smaller one. Since the formula for the mean takes sample size into account by dividing the summed X values by N, it is unnecessary to introduce any changes into the numerator of the standardized score formula when working with samples of unequal size.

When comparing related samples, such as data from one group of subjects measured at two points in time, the researcher computes a single standard deviation based on the *difference* between the first and second measurements. Table 11.3 presents hypothetical data on eight subjects measured at two points in time. The standard deviation for these data can be computed by using the formula:

$$\sigma = \sqrt{\frac{\Sigma D^2}{N} - (\overline{X}_1 - \overline{X}_2)^2} \qquad (11.7)$$

where σ = standard deviation of before and after difference scores

D = remainder when value for second observation is subtracted from value for first observation

N = number of subjects in sample

Once the standard deviation has been found, it is then possible to calculate the standard error of the difference by using the following formula:

$$\sigma_{\text{diff}} = \frac{\sigma}{\sqrt{N}} \qquad (11.8)$$

where σ = standard deviation of the difference scores

N = number of subjects in the sample

The resulting σ_{diff} is then substituted into the denominator of the formula for the t value. The numerator contains the mean of the first measure $(\overline{X}_1)$ minus the mean of the second measure $(\overline{X}_2)$. Table 11.3 demonstrates this process. It is important to note that, when working with related samples, the degree of freedom equals $N - 1$. N stands for the total number of *cases* (each measured twice) and not for the total number of scores. Thus the degree of freedom equals 7 in this example.

To see if it would be possible to reject a null hypothesis that no difference exists between the first and second measurements of the group in favor of a research hypothesis that a difference does exist, we must compare the computed t value of -5.09 with the minimum t value needed to reject H_0. Assuming that we have set our level of significance at .05 and that we have stated a nondirectional research hypothesis, this minimum value is ± 2.365 when we are working with 7 degrees of freedom. Since our calculated t score of -5.09 exceeds this minimum, we reject H_0. Had we stated a directional hypothesis and predicted that the mean at the first measurement would be less than the mean at the second measurement $(\overline{X}_1 < \overline{X}_2)$, we would have needed a minimum t value of -1.895 to reject H_0.

Restrictions on the Use of Difference-Between-Means Tests

In addition to the assumptions stated at the beginning of this chapter, the greatest restriction of the t test is that it restricts

Table 11.3. Steps in Calculating a *t* Value for Related Samples

Subject	X_1 First measure	X_2 Second measure	$X_1 - X_2$ Difference	D^2 Difference squared
1	4	8	−4	16
2	2	4	−2	4
3	6	12	−6	36
4	9	18	−9	81
5	2	4	−2	4
6	8	16	−8	64
7	4	8	−4	16
8	2	4	−2	4
	$\Sigma X_1 = 37$	$\Sigma X_2 = 74$		$\Sigma D^2 = 225$

Step 1: Calculate $\overline{X}_1$ and $\overline{X}_2$ ($\overline{X} = \dfrac{\Sigma fX}{N}$)

$$\overline{X}_1 = \frac{37}{8}$$

$$= 4.62$$

$$\overline{X}_2 = \frac{74}{8}$$

$$= 9.25$$

Step 2: Calculate standard deviation for difference between first measure and second measure

$$\sigma = \sqrt{\frac{\Sigma D^2}{N} - (\overline{X}_1 - \overline{X}_2)^2}$$

$$\sigma = \sqrt{\frac{225}{8} - (4.62 - 9.25)^2}$$

$$= \sqrt{28.12 - (-4.63)^2}$$

$$= \sqrt{28.12 - 21.44}$$

$$= \sqrt{6.68}$$

$$= 2.58$$

Step 3: Calculate standard error of difference

$$\sigma_{\text{diff}} = \frac{\sigma}{\sqrt{N}}$$

$$\sigma_{\text{diff}} = \frac{2.58}{\sqrt{8}}$$

$$= \frac{2.58}{2.83}$$

$$= .91$$

Step 4: Calculate standardized score

$$t = \frac{\overline{X}_1 - \overline{X}_2}{\sigma_{\text{diff}}}$$

$$t = \frac{4.62 - 9.25}{.91}$$

$$= \frac{-4.63}{.91}$$

$$= -5.09$$

the user to the comparison of only two groups. Many times the researcher is interested in comparing three or more groups. For example, there are numerous studies comparing diploma, associate, and baccalaureate graduates in nursing. In such cases an analysis of variance (ANOVA) is applied to the data. The technique allows the researcher to determine if the amount of variation (variance) *between* the groups being compared exceeds the amount of variation *within* each group. If it can be demonstrated that the variation between groups is significantly greater than that within groups, this will support a research hypothesis that the comparison groups significantly differ from one another. This is done by converting the raw data to a standardized score called an *F ratio* and using the *F* distribution to interpret the results. While we will not actually calculate an *F* ratio, it is important for the student to be aware of its existence and to have a general understanding of how it is interpreted.[6]

Reference

Gorman, J.   A prospective study of the merits of circoelectric vs. the standard hospital bed in the post-operative management of spinal-cord fusions for scoliosis. Unpublished manuscript, 1978.

WORKING WITH AND INTERPRETING DATA

1. Refer again to the data comparing when La Leche League members and nonmembers first introduced solid foods into their child's diet (Chapter 3, problem 2). Apply the *t* test to these data to test the following research hypothesis: La Leche League members introduce solid foods into their child's diet later than nonmembers, $H_1 : \overline{X}_1 > \overline{X}_2$.

2. You have now applied a chi-square test, median test, and *t* test to the same data (introduction of solid foods). Compare the results of all three tests. Discuss the relative appropriateness and usefulness of each.

3. The following scores come from a random sample of students in our statistics course. They are students' scores on the first and second examination of the quarter in which the sample was drawn. Use the appropriate *t* test to test the following research hypothesis: Student scores on the first examination differ significantly from their scores on the second examination.

[6] For a complete discussion of analysis of variance, see Loether and McTavish (1974b, pp. 176-186).

Student	Exam 1 Scores	Exam 2 Scores
1	95	68
2	90	86
3	95	59
4	95	86
5	90	78
6	87	71
7	98	89
8	90	79
9	90	65
10	100	42
11	90	94
12	75	53
13	100	59
14	95	78
15	95	66

4. Indicate whether the following t test values are significant or non-significant:

   a. $H_1 : \overline{X}_1 \neq \overline{X}_2$

   $N_1 = 15$

   $N_2 = 15$

   $\alpha = .05$

   $t = 2.50$

   b. $H_1 : \overline{X}_1 > \overline{X}_2$

   $N_1 = 20$

   $N_2 = 10$

   $\alpha = .01$

   $t = 2.03$

   c. $H_1 : \overline{X}_1 < \overline{X}_2$

   $N_1 = 12$

   $N_2 = 14$

   $\alpha = .05$

   $t = 1.93$

5. The authors of the following articles analyze data by using a t test. For each article, describe and interpret the author's findings. Evaluate the appropriateness of their use of the t test, paying special attention to the appropriateness of the specific t test that the author has used.

Godejohn, Carol J., Jacqueline Taylor, Ann F. Muhlen-kamp, and Willard Blaesser. Effect of simulation gaming on attitudes toward mental illness. *Nursing Research* 24:367, 1975.

Lindeman, Carol A., and Betty Van Aernam. Nursing intervention with the presurgical patient—the effects of structured and unstructured preoperative teaching. *Nursing Research* 20:319, 1971.

Muhlenkamp, Ann F., Lucille D. Gress, and Mary A. Flood. Perceptions of life change events by the elderly. *Nursing Research* 24:109, 1975.

Relationships Between Two Variables

III

Measures of Association

In practice, few if any events occur in total isolation. They are almost always the result of the joint operation of at least two factors. Therefore in addition to describing how observations are distributed for a single variable, researchers are also interested in analyzing the distribution of observations for two variables simultaneously. In other words the researcher wishes to investigate whether two variables are *related* to one another in some way. For example, in a study of patient mortality a researcher might examine whether death due to lung cancer is related to cigarette smoking; another researcher studying the problems of patients with chronic disabilities might examine whether certain problems are related to the patient's age.

As presented in Chapter 9, one approach to such an analysis problem is to test whether the occurrence of an observation in a particular category of one variable is contingent upon the category in which that same observation occurs for another variable, by the application of the chi-square test, for example. However, while tests of contingency indicate whether a relationship *exists* between two variables, they give no indication regarding two extremely important aspects of a relationship: direction and strength. The *direction* of a relationship refers to whether one variable increases if the other increases (a positive relationship) or whether it decreases when the other increases (a negative relationship). The *strength* of a relationship refers to how reliably the amount of change in one variable may be predicted given an observed change of a certain amount in the other variable. It is of minimal use to either the researcher or the clinical practitioner to know that a relationship exists between two variables without also knowing the nature or direction and strength of the relationship.

Statistics that indicate the direction and/or strength of a relationship are collectively referred to as *measures of association*. After a discussion of the basic characteristics of measures of association, this chapter will introduce the *proportional reduction in error* approach to measuring association, which will then be applied in the presentation of four measures of association: lambda, for nominal level variables, and gamma, Somers' d, and Kendall's tau for ordinal level variables. Relationships between two interval level variables will be discussed in the next chapter.

Characteristics of Measures of Association

Three aspects of a distribution of bivariate observations (that is, observations made on two variables simultaneously) are of interest in a statistical analysis. The first aspect is whether a relationship exists between the two variables. If no relationship is apparent, the analysis need proceed no farther. If a relationship is present, however, it then remains to describe its direction and strength. For convenience in interpretation, there are certain conventions that a measure of association should follow.

EXISTENCE OF A RELATIONSHIP
A measure of association should equal a value of zero when no relationship exists.

DIRECTION OF A RELATIONSHIP
The direction of a relationship should be indicated by the arithmetic sign of the measure of association: a positive sign for a positive relationship (as one variable increases, so does the other); a negative sign for a negative relationship (as one variable increases, the other decreases). It should be obvious that it is not possible to consider the direction of a relationship between nominal level variables, because only the ordinal and interval levels of measurement reflect the ordering of observations along the measurement scale.

A familiar example of a positive relationship is that between age and weight in children: As a child becomes older, he or she tends to weigh more. On the other hand there may be a negative relationship between surgical patients' preoperative stress levels and postoperative recovery rates. That is, postoperative recovery rates tend to be high among patients who experience low preoperative stress and low among patients who experience high preoperative stress.

STRENGTH OF A RELATIONSHIP
The size or magnitude of a measure of association should indicate the strength of a relationship. If a value of zero indicates no relationship, the farther from zero the value of a measure of association is, the stronger is the relationship. Furthermore, the value of a measure of association should be limited within a fixed range of possible values between zero and some maximum. This is so that the strength of a relationship may be evaluated in terms of how close it is to the strongest relationship possible: the closer the value of a measure of association to the maximum possible value, the stronger the relationship. It is especially desirable that a measure of association be standardized so that its maximum possible value is 1.00, because this greatly facilitates the interpretation of the strength of a relationship according to the value of the measure of association by confining it within a convenient and well-defined range of possible values. Thus, for most measures of association a value of $+1.00$ indicates a

maximum positive relationship while a value of -1.00 indicates a maximum negative relationship.

Association vs. Contingency

In order to illustrate the advantage of measures of association over measures of contingency, let us consider the relationship between smoking and death due to lung cancer. As presented in Table 12.1, there is a positive relationship between these two variables, with a greater chance of death due to lung cancer among smokers (90%) than among nonsmokers (20%). The existence of this relationship is indicated by the chi-square value, which is significant at the .01 level.

Now consider the relationship between smoking and death due to lung cancer as presented in Table 12.2. This table was derived by simply taking the observations that appear in the first column of Table 12.1 and placing them in the second column of Table 12.2, and taking the observations from the second column of Table 12.1 and placing them in the first column of Table 12.2. The result of this reversal of the position of the observations in Table 12.2 is a reversal in the relationship between smoking and death due to lung cancer (although this is unrealistic, it will help to illustrate an

Table 12.1. Incidence of Death Due to Lung Cancer, by Smoking Behavior

Death due to lung cancer?	Smoking behavior (number of subjects in parentheses)	
	Nonsmoker	Smoker
No	80% (16)	10% (2)
Yes	20% (4)	90% (18)
Total	100% (20)	100% (20)

$\chi^2 = 19.78$; df $= 1$; $p < .01$

Table 12.2. Incidence of Death Due to Lung Cancer, by Smoking Behavior

Death due to lung cancer?	Smoking behavior (number of subjects in parentheses)	
	Nonsmoker	Smoker
No	10% (2)	80% (16)
Yes	90% (18)	20% (4)
Total	100% (20)	100% (20)

$\chi^2 = 19.78$; df $= 1$; $p < .01$

important point). That is, as displayed in Table 12.2, there is a greater chance of death due to lung cancer among the non-smokers (90%) than among the smokers (20%). The existence of this relationship is also indicated by a chi-square value that is significant at the .01 level.

Although the relationship in Table 12.2 is the exact opposite of that in Table 12.1, however, the chi-square values calculated for these tables are identical in both sign and magnitude. If we had not examined the percentage distributions within these tables, we would have been misled into thinking that they displayed identical relationships. Thus a major disadvantage of the chi-square test is that it will always have a positive value and cannot indicate whether the direction of a relationship is positive or negative.

The fact that the size of the chi-square value (19.78) is the same for both tables suggests that we compare chi-square values to determine the relative strength of a relationship. That is, because the chi-square values are equal in this case, we might conclude that the relationships are equally strong. On the other hand, if one value were larger than the other, we might conclude that the table with the larger chi-square value displayed a stronger relationship. Thus, because the chi-square for Table 12.3 (197.98) is larger than that for Table 12.1, we might conclude that the relationship displayed in Table 12.3 is stronger than that in Table 12.1. Furthermore it would appear logical to conclude that, because the chi-square value for Table 12.3 is ten times larger than that for Table 12.1, the strength of the relationship in Table 12.3 is ten times that in Table 12.1. But this conclusion would be *incorrect*.

It would be incorrect because the value of a chi-square test is related to the total number of observations in the table for which it is computed. The larger the total number of observations, the larger the chi-square value may be. Thus the chi-square value for Table 12.3 is ten times that for Table 12.1 because the total number of observations in Table 12.3

Table 12.3. Incidence of Death Due to Lung Cancer, by Smoking Behavior

Death due to lung cancer?	Smoking behavior (number of subjects in parentheses)	
	Nonsmoker	Smoker
No	80% (160)	10% (20)
Yes	20% (40)	90% (180)
Total	100% (200)	100% (200)

$\chi^2 = 197.98$; df $= 1$; $p < .01$

($N=400$) is ten times that for Table 12.1 ($N=40$) and not because of a difference in the strength of the relationships they display. In fact an examination of the percentage distributions within Tables 12.1 and 12.3 reveals identical positive relationships, with smokers being more likely to die due to lung cancer (90%) than nonsmokers (20%) in both tables.

Also, chi-square values may not be compared between tables with different degrees of freedom. The reason for this is apparent from examination of Table C.3 in Appendix C. Critical values of chi-square, at any given level of significance, increase as the degrees of freedom increase. In fact there is no maximum value for a chi-square test, which may range from zero to infinity.[1] In general, for a relationship of a given strength, the chi-square value increases as the degrees of freedom increases. Therefore a comparison of chi-square values for two tables is appropriate only in the rather infrequent situation in which the total number of observations and degrees of freedom are the same.

Thus a chi-square value may not be interpreted as indicating either the direction or the strength of a relationship.

Asymmetrical and Symmetrical Measures of Association

Measures of association may be grouped into two broad categories according to the way they are computed and interpreted. *Asymmetrical* measures of association indicate how useful knowledge is about an independent variable (X) in predicting categories or values of a dependent variable (Y). It is possible to compute two different values of an asymmetrical measure for a single bivariate distribution by alternately considering each variable as the independent and as the dependent variable. Thus we may compute a measure for the relationship when variable X is considered as the independent variable ($X \to Y$) and when variable Y is considered as the independent variable ($X \leftarrow Y$).

Symmetrical measures of association do not distinguish between independent and dependent variables. These measures indicate the degree to which changes in each of two variables *coincide* with one another. An observed change in variable Y, for example, may be either a cause or an effect of a change in variable X, and vice versa. Furthermore it is also possible that both variables X and Y change simultaneously in reaction to a change in a third variable (Z):

[1] There is measure of contingency, called *Cramer's V*, which may be interpreted as indicating the strength of a relationship. Cramer's V, computed as $V = \sqrt{\chi^2/Nt}$, where t is the smaller of the two quantities $(R-1)$ or $(C-1)$, may be interpreted as a standardized chi-square because the value of V may range from zero to $+1.00$. See Loether and McTavish, 1974a, for a detailed discussion.

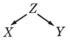

Thus, the observed relationship between variables X and Y may be coincidental to their mutual dependence upon the independent variable Z.

The distinction between asymmetrical and symmetrical measures of association is an important consideration in deciding which measure is the most appropriate for a particular analysis situation. Both asymmetrical and symmetrical measures will be presented in this and the following chapter.

Selection of an Appropriate Measure of Association

Many different measures of association may be used to describe a relationship between two variables. The decision as to which measure is the most appropriate for any given analysis situation depends primarily upon two factors: the level of measurement of each variable and the purpose of the analysis.

Each measure of association requires a particular minimum level of measurement for each variable. For example, while some measures may be used for two variables that are both measured at the nominal level (or higher), some require that at least one of the variables be measured at either the ordinal or the interval level, and others require that both variables be measured at either the ordinal or the interval level.

Furthermore each measure of association is designed to provide a unique kind of information about the relationship being analyzed. Therefore, as in the case of selecting a measure of central tendency, the researcher must select a measure that will provide the information necessary to answer the research question under study. Although many technical considerations may be considered in this regard, the most important question is whether an asymmetrical or a symmetrical measure is required. If the researcher wishes to examine a causal relationship, then an asymmetrical measure should be selected, while a symmetrical measure should be selected when the researcher wishes to discover whether changes in each of two variables tend to coincide.

There are many different measures of association, and it is impossible for most people to remember exactly how each one is computed and interpreted. Given the kinds of data and research questions with which researchers work most often, however, only a relatively small number of measures of association are used frequently. Use of the others is reserved for analysis situations for which they are especially designed. It is sufficient for a researcher to know that these special purpose measures exist and what references to consult when it is necessary to compute and/or interpret one.

To simplify the situation further, Costner (1965) described a common logical system for intuitively understanding the computation and interpretation of most of the measures of association that are used most often. This system, discussed in the following section, is called the *proportional reduction in error* approach and will be applied to each of the measures of association presented in this chapter. It will also be applied in the discussion of correlation in Chapter 13.

Proportional Reduction in Error Measures

If two variables are related to each other, then information about each of the two variables should generally be more useful than information about either of them alone. Measures of association that follow the proportional reduction in error (PRE) approach indicate how much more useful information about two variables is than information about only one of them. In other words, the main focus of this approach is to examine the degree to which one variable is able to account for, or explain, variation among observations on another variable.

To the extent that a researcher is able to explain variation on a given variable (Y), he or she will be successful in predicting categories or values of observations on that variable when provided with some information that describes the distribution of observations on that variable. Of course prediction errors will also be experienced to the extent that the researcher is not able to explain all the variation on that variable. But rather than stop at this point, the researcher may collect additional information about the same set of observations regarding a second variable (X), which he or she believes is related to the first variable. If there is in fact a relationship between the two variables, then this additional information should enable the researcher to further explain variation among observations on the first variable. Using information about variable X, the researcher should make fewer prediction errors regarding categories or values of observations on variable Y than previously.

COMPUTATION

A convenient method for measuring the reduction in prediction errors is to compute the proportion of errors committed using information about variable Y only that are eliminated by the addition of information about variable X. Thus the researcher may compute a measure of association that is interpreted as the proportional *reduction* in errors committed in predicting categories or values of one variable when knowledge about the distribution of observations on another variable is added.

The PRE method of measuring association between two variables consists of four elements:

Prediction Rule 1. A rule for predicting categories or values of a variable (Y) on the basis of knowledge about the distribution of observations on that variable only.
Errors Committed Using Rule 1 (E_1). A method of measuring prediction errors committed when prediction rule 1 is applied.
Prediction Rule 2. A rule for predicting categories or values of a variable (Y) with the addition of knowledge about the distribution of observations on a second variable (X).
Errors Committed Using Rule 2 (E_2). A method for measuring prediction errors committed when prediction rule 2 is applied.

The specific statement of each prediction rule and method of measuring prediction errors is different for each PRE measure of association. As will be seen in the discussion of the PRE measures presented in this book, these statements are dependent upon the level of measurement of the variables and the purpose of the analysis.

The general computational format of all PRE measures is

$$\text{PRE} = \frac{E_1 - E_2}{E_1} \qquad (12.1)$$

When variable X is not related to variable Y, the researcher's ability to predict categories or values of variable Y will not improve with knowledge of variable X. Under this condition, therefore, prediction errors committed using rule 1 (E_1) will not be reduced, and prediction errors committed using rule 2 (E_2) will equal those for rule 1. The fact that there is no relationship between variables X and Y will be indicated by a value of zero for the PRE measure, as indicated below.

when $E_2 = E_1$

$$\text{PRE} = \frac{E_1 - E_2}{E_1} = \frac{E_1 - E_1}{E_1} = \frac{0}{E_1} = 0$$

If there is a perfect positive relationship between variables X and Y, prediction rule 2 will enable the researcher to predict perfectly for all categories or values of variable Y. Therefore *all* prediction errors committed when rule 1 is used will be eliminated, and *no* prediction errors will be committed when prediction rule 2 is used. Under this condition the PRE measure will equal $+1.00$.

when $E_2 = 0$

$$\text{PRE} = \frac{E_1 - E_2}{E_1} = \frac{E_1 - 0}{E_1} = \frac{E_1}{E_1} = +1.00$$

While it is not difficult to understand how and why a PRE measure will equal zero when there is no relationship, and $+1.00$ when there is a perfect positive relationship, the explanation of why a value of -1.00 will be obtained when there is a perfect negative relationship is somewhat abstract at this point. It will become clearer when the computation of specific PRE measures is discussed in the following sections.

Mathematically a PRE measure will equal -1.00 when $E_2 = 2E_1$. That is, twice as many prediction errors must be committed when rule 2 is used as when rule 1 is used.

when $E_2 = 2E_1$

$$\text{PRE} = \frac{E_1 - E_2}{E_1} = \frac{E_1 - 2E_1}{E_1} = \frac{-E_1}{E_1} = -1.00$$

But this does not seem to make sense at first, because we want to *reduce* prediction errors, not increase them! It must be recognized however, that, because it is not possible to make predictions in two opposite directions at the same time, prediction rule 2 is always stated on the assumption that there is a positive relationship between the variables. Thus, if predictions are made in a positive direction and the actual relationship is negative, then more errors will be committed than if no assumption were made regarding the direction of the relationship, as is the case when prediction rule 1 is applied. This is illustrated in Table 12.4 in which "O" indicates the cell location of the observed categories or values for both X and Y, which are negatively related. The cell location of the predicted categories or values of Y, indicated by "P," assume a positive relationship and are completely in error.

Table 12.4. Observed (O) and Predicted (P) Cell Locations for a Negative PRE Measure

| | Variable X | | | |
Variable Y	Very low	Low	High	Very high
Very low	P			O
Low		P	O	
High		O	P	
Very high	O			P

However, if the predictions had been made in the correct direction (negative in this case), *no* prediction errors would have been committed.

In summary, if the same number of errors are committed using rule 2 as using rule 1, then the variables are not related, because knowledge about variable X does not improve our ability to predict categories or values of variable Y. The PRE measure will equal zero. To the extent that there is a positive relationship between variables X and Y, fewer prediction errors will be committed using rule 2 than rule 1, and the value of the PRE measure will be positive and greater than zero, with a value of $+1.00$ indicating a perfect positive relationship. To the extent that there is a negative relationship between variables X and Y, more prediction errors will be committed using rule 2 than rule 1, and the value of the PRE measure will be negative, with a value of -1.00 indicating a perfect negative relationship.

INTERPRETATION

The arithmetic sign, plus or minus, of a PRE measure indicates, whether the direction of a relationship is positive or negative. The absolute value of a PRE measure indicates the proportion of prediction errors committed using prediction rule 1 that are eliminated by switching to prediction rule 2. Because prediction rule 1 is based upon knowledge about the distribution of observations on one variable (Y) only, while rule 2 is based upon additional knowledge about the distribution of observations on another variable (X), variable X may be considered as explaining variation on variable Y to the extent that it contributes to a reduction in prediction errors. Thus the size of a PRE measure may be interpreted as indicating the percentage of variation in variable Y that is explained by variable X. Caution must be exercised in using this interpretation, however, because in a very strict sense it is appropriate only for asymmetrical measures in the analysis of causal relationships. That is, a symmetrical PRE measure may also be appropriately interpreted as indicating the percentage of variation in variable X that is explained by variable Y.

Figure 12.1 is presented as a general guide to evaluating the strength of a relationship as indicated by a PRE measure. A researcher would like to explain at least 50 percent of the variance in most cases. Therefore a PRE measure of .50 is often used as the cut-off point to distinguish a weak relationship from a strong one. Each researcher must decide for him- or herself where an appropriate cut-off point is, however, depending on the quality of the data and the purpose of the

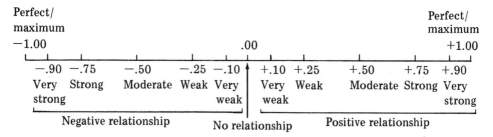

Figure 12.1. Guide to evaluating strength of PRE measures of association.

analysis. That is, when exploring an area in which little or no research has been conducted previously, and/or valid and reliable measurement methods have not been developed, it would be wise for the researcher not to ignore relatively weak relationships because these may indicate areas that warrant more concentrated investigation in the future. On the other hand, when conducting research in an area in which a considerable amount of research has been already reported and/or when using measurement methods whose validity and reliability are well established, the researcher may be more demanding of the findings and focus only on relationships that are relatively strong and that appear the most worthwhile investigating in future research.

Also, as will be discussed in the following sections, each PRE measure must also be tested for statistical significance. Regardless of how large a measure of association is, it is meaningless if it is not statistically significant, because it is likely to be the result of chance. When the statistical significance of a measure of association is tested, the null hypothesis is that there is no relationship between the two variables. In other words, the null hypothesis states that the measure of association does not significantly differ from zero.

Lambda
Lambda (λ) is an asymmetrical PRE measure of association between two nominal level variables. Although it can also be computed for ordinal or interval level variables, it is more appropriate to use other measures to deal with those variables. Furthermore, because lambda is designed especially for nominal level variables, which do not display directionality in their relationships, its value will always be positive, ranging from 0 to +1.00.

COMPUTATION

Following the PRE format, the prediction rules and definitions of error for lambda may be generally stated as follows.

Prediction Rule 1: Predict the modal category of the dependent variable for every observation.

Errors Committed Using Rule 1 (E_1): Find the number of
observations that are not located within the modal category
of the dependent variable.

Prediction Rule 2: Predict the modal category of the dependent variable within each category of the independent
variable.

Errors Committed Using Rule 2 (E_2): Find the total number
of observations that are not located within the modal category of the dependent variable within each category of the
independent variable.

The computational formula for lambda is[2]

$$\lambda = \frac{(N - f_{md}) - \Sigma(n_i - f_{mi})}{N - f_{md}} \qquad (12.2)$$

where λ = lambda

f_{md} = number of observations located within the modal
category of the dependent variable

f_{mi} = number of observations located within the modal
category of the dependent variable within each
category of the independent variable

n_i = total number of observations located within each
category of the independent variable

N = total number of observations

Note that $E_1 = N - f_{md}$, $E_2 = \Sigma(n_i - f_{mi})$, and therefore
formula 12.2 follows the general PRE format:

$$\lambda = \frac{E_1 - E_2}{E_1}$$

We may now compute a value of lambda for the relationship between smoking and death due to lung cancer presented in Table 12.5, treating "death due to lung cancer" as

[2] An alternative computation formula is

$$\lambda = \frac{\Sigma f_{mi} - f_{md}}{N - f_{md}}$$

For the purposes of this book, this formula is not preferred, because it
does not follow PRE format and provides only a very slight computational advantage.

Table 12.5. Incidence of Death Due to Lung Cancer, by Smoking Behavior

| Death due to lung cancer? | Smoking Behavior | | Total |
	Nonsmoker	Smoker	
No	16	2	18
Yes	4	18	22
Total	20	20	40

the dependent variable. Given only the frequency distribution for death due to lung cancer, the best we could do in attempting to predict whether any one of the 40 individuals died due to lung cancer would be to predict the modal category "Yes" for all cases. Accordingly we would commit 18 prediction errors ($E_1 = N - f_{md} = 40 - 22 = 18$). But once we were told that an individual was a nonsmoker, we would be most successful if we predicted the modal category "No" for all cases within that category of the independent variable ("smoking behavior"), committing 4 prediction errors ($n_i - f_{mi} = 20 - 16 = 4$). On the other hand, if we knew that an individual was a smoker, we would be most successful if we predicted the modal category "Yes" for all cases within that category of the independent variable, committing 2 prediction errors ($n_i - f_{mi} = 20 - 18 = 2$). Thus the total number of prediction errors that would be committed with the addition of knowledge about the distribution of the 40 individuals regarding smoking behavior is 6 [($E_2 = \Sigma(n_i - f_{mi}) = 4 + 2 = 6$)]. Computing a value of lambda according to formula 12.2, we obtain the result:

$$\lambda = \frac{(N - f_{md}) - \Sigma(n_i - f_{mi})}{N - f_{md}} = \frac{18 - (4 + 2)}{18}$$

$$= \frac{18 - 6}{18} = \frac{12}{18} = .67$$

INTERPRETATION

The value .67 obtained for lambda for Table 12.5 indicates that 67 percent of the prediction errors that were initially committed using knowledge only about the distribution of observations according to death due to lung cancer were reduced or eliminated by the addition of knowledge about how the observations were also distributed according to smoking behavior. In other words, smoking behavior explains 67 percent of the variation for death due to lung cancer in this example.

This indicates that there is a moderate to strong relationship between smoking and death due to lung cancer, with death due to lung cancer being least likely among nonsmokers and most likely among smokers. Note, however, that the nature of this relationship must be derived by visual examination of Table 12.5. It is important to remember that, because the value of lambda will always be positive, it is not possible to determine the nature of a relationship by examination of a lambda value. Although this is not a serious drawback when dealing with nominal level variables, where the concept of directionality of relationship (in terms of positive and negative) is not applicable, it is the main reason why lambda is not an appropriate measure of association when both variables are measured at the ordinal or higher level.

SIGNIFICANCE

The procedure for testing the statistical significance of lambda is complex and therefore will not be presented here.[3] A crude but useful test of the significance of lambda may be obtained by computing a chi-square value for the relationship being examined. In general, if the chi-square value is significant, it may be assumed that the value of lambda is also significant. One should be cautious about making this assumption when the chi-square value is only slightly larger than the critical value at the designated alpha level, however, because the risk of committing a type I error may be increased. That is, the lambda value may not be significant although the chi-square value is.

For example, the significance of the value of lambda that was computed for the relationship in Table 12.5 may be tested by referring to the chi-square value for the same data set in Table 12.1. Because that chi-square value was found to be significant at the .01 level, it may be concluded that the value of lambda is also significant.

A NOTE ON ASYMMETRY

In the case of Table 12.5 it would not be logical to compute a value of lambda treating smoking behavior as the dependent variable and death due to lung cancer as the independent variable because death due to lung cancer is not antecedent to smoking behavior. However, it is not mathematically impossible to compute a value of lambda for that condition. If this were done, the following result would be obtained:

$$\lambda = \frac{(N - f_{md}) - \Sigma(n_i - f_{mi})}{N - f_{md}} = \frac{(40 - 20) - (2 + 4)}{40 - 20}$$

$$= \frac{20 - 6}{20} = \frac{14}{20} = .70$$

It is important to note that this is not the same result that was obtained when death due to lung cancer was treated as the

---

[3] Interested readers should see Reynolds (1977, p. 50).

dependent variable. Therefore one must be careful to distinguish clearly between the dependent and independent variable whenever calculating an asymmetrical measure of association.

MEASURING ASSOCIATION BETWEEN A NOMINAL AND A HIGHER LEVEL VARIABLE

Lambda is an appropriate measure of association even when one of the variables is measured at either the ordinal or interval level, as long as the other variable is nominal. Furthermore it does not matter whether the nominal level variable is designated as the independent or the dependent variable. For example, a value of lambda may be computed for the relationship between three different nursing interventions and patient evaluations of the quality of nursing care, as presented in Table 12.6. Treating quality of nursing care as the dependent variable, lambda is computed as

$$\lambda = \frac{(N - f_{md}) - \Sigma(n_i - f_{mi})}{N - f_{md}} = \frac{(115 - 45) - (25 + 15 + 22)}{115 - 45}$$

$$= \frac{70 - 62}{70} = \frac{8}{70} = .11$$

Although this result is statistically significant ($x^2 = 11.79$; df $= 4$; $p < .05$), it indicates only a weak relationship.

Gamma

Gamma (γ) (also referred to as *Goodman and Kruskal's G*) is a symmetrical proportional reduction in error measure of association between two ordinal level variables. Its value may range from -1.00 to $+1.00$. It is useful to think of gamma as a member of a family of ordinal level, PRE measures of association because of its close similarity to two other measures that will be discussed in the following sections, Somers' *d* and Kendall's tau. The numerator of the computational formula is exactly the same for all three of these measures. Their denominators differ slightly, depending on which of several

Table 12.6. Nursing Intervention and Patient Evaluation of Quality of Nursing Care

Nursing intervention	Patient evaluation of quality of nursing care			Total
	Poor	*Fair*	*Good*	*Total*
Method A	12	13	15	40
Method B	5	10	21	36
Method C	17	13	9	39
Total	34	36	45	115

assumptions the researcher is willing to make. Therefore the discussions of Somers' d and Kendall's tau will require only relatively simple extensions of the discussion of gamma.

The computation of gamma focuses on the examination of pairs of observations. For example, in a study of the relationship between perceived severity of a particular health problem and compliance with a prescribed regimen, an observation may be the finding that a patient perceives a low degree of severity and displays a medium degree of compliance. This can be symbolized, as shown in Table 12.7, by "LM," where variable X is perceived severity and variable Y is compliance. All cases of patients found to perceive a low degree of severity and found to display a medium degree of compliance are included in the cell labeled "LM." A *pair* of observations may be identified, for example, as consisting of a patient included in the "LM" cell and a patient included in the "MH" cell (a medium degree of perceived severity and a high degree of compliance). Each observation in a data set is paired with *every* other observation, one at a time, to compare their relative rankings on each of two ordinal variables. For example, in Table 12.7 each LM observation may be paired for comparison with each other LM observation, and with each LL observation, and with each MH observation, and so on. When rankings are compared, it is found, for example, that in an "LM and MH" pair variable X is low for the first observation and medium for the second observation; variable Y is medium for the first observation and high for the second observation. In this particular pair, the second observation ranks relatively higher than the first observation for both variables X and Y.

Three basic types of pairs may be identified for two variables: tied pairs, same-ordered pairs, and reverse-ordered pairs. These will be described by referring to the schematic illustration in Table 12.7. It is important to note that the categories for both ordinal variables, X and Y, are arranged so that they are ordered from low to high, originating at the upper left-hand corner of the table. The arrangement of observations in this way is vital for the computation of gamma as shown here.

TIED PAIRS
A pair of observations is considered to be *tied* when both observations in the pair have the same ranking on one or both

Table 12.7. Schematic Illustration of Bivariate Ordinal Observations

	Variable Y		
Variable X	Low	Medium	High
Low	LL	LM	LH
Medium	ML	MM	MH
High	HL	HM	HH

variables. For example, each of the observations located in the cell labeled "LM" in Table 12.7 may be compared with each of the observations that fall in the same category on variable X (low) but in a different category on variable Y (low and high). These observations are located in the cells labeled "LL" and "LH" respectively. Although there are differences among these pairs of observations regarding their ranking on variable Y, they all have the same ranking on variable X and are therefore considered to be tied on variable X.

Similarly, each of the LM observations may be compared with each of the observations that fall in a different category on variable X (medium and high) but the same category on variable Y (medium). These observations are located in the cells labeled "MM" and "HM" respectively. Although these pairs of observations differ regarding their ranking on variable X, they all have the same ranking on variable Y and are considered to be tied on variable Y.

Furthermore, each of the LM observations may be compared with every other observation located within the LM cell. Because they all have the same ranking on both variables X and Y, that is, they are all low on variable X and medium on variable Y, they are considered to be tied on both variables.

In other words, each observation is tied on variable X with every other observation that is located within the same row of Table 12.7; each observation is tied on variable Y with every other observation that is located within the same column of the table; and each observation is tied on both variables X and Y with every other observation that is located within the same cell of the table. The location of all tied pairs that include the LM observations is illustrated in Table 12.8.

Because gamma is a measure of our ability to make predictions regarding *ordered* pairs, all tied pairs are excluded in the computation of gamma. It is important to be able to identify tied pairs not only to exclude them from the computation of gamma but also because certain kinds of tied pairs are *included* in the computation of Somers' d and Kendall's tau.

SAME-ORDERED PAIRS

The ordering of a pair of observations is considered to be the *same* when the ranking of one observation is lower than the

Table 12.8. Location of Tied Pairs That Include LM Observations

Variable X	Variable Y		
	Low	Medium	High
Low	LL	LM	LH
Medium	ML	MM	MH
High	HL	HM	HH

other on *both* variables. For example, an LM observation is lower on both variable X and variable Y than any observation that is located in the cells labeled "MH" and "HH." As a rule of thumb, the same-ordered pairs that include the observations in any given cell may be found by pairing each observation in that cell with each observation in all cells that are located *below and to the right* of that cell. This is illustrated in Table 12.9 and demonstrates the importance of arranging the categories as suggested in Table 12.7.

REVERSE-ORDERED PAIRS
The ordering of a pair of observations is considered to be *reversed* when the ranking of one observation is lower than the other on one variable and higher than the other on the other variable. For example, an LM observation is *lower* on variable X than any observation located in the cells labeled "ML" and "HL." However, an LM observation is *higher* on variable Y than an ML and HL observation. As a rule of thumb, the reverse-ordered pairs that include the observations in any given cell may be found by pairing each observation in that cell with each observation in all cells that are located *below and to the left* of that cell. This is illustrated in Table 12.10.

COMPUTATION
The conceptual formula for the computation of gamma follows the PRE format. However, because that formula is not efficient in practice, a simplified computational formula is

Table 12.9. Location of Same-Ordered Pairs That Include LM Observations

| Variable X | | Variable Y | |
	Low	Medium	High
Low	LL	(LM)	LH
Medium	ML	MM	MH
High	HL	HM	HH

Table 12.10. Location of Reverse-Ordered Pairs That Include LM Observations

| Variable X | | Variable Y | |
	Low	Medium	High
Low	LL	(LM)	LH
Medium	ML	MM	MH
High	HL	HM	HH

presented following a discussion of the conceptual approach.

Gamma indicates the relative preponderance of same- and reverse-ordered pairs of observations. In order to understand what this means, let us consider some possible relationships. For example, Table 12.11 illustrates the pattern that would be observed if there were a perfect *positive* relationship between variables X and Y. All ordered pairs in this situation are *same-ordered*; there are no reverse-ordered pairs. The computed value of gamma for such a pattern would equal + 1.00. Gamma will be positive whenever there are more same-ordered than reverse-ordered pairs.

On the other hand gamma will equal − 1.00 when observations are distributed in the pattern displayed in Table 12.12, which illustrates a perfect *negative* relationship between variables X and Y. In this situation all ordered pairs are *reverse-ordered*; there are no same-ordered pairs. Gamma will be negative whenever there are more reverse-ordered than same-ordered pairs.

Finally, gamma will equal .00, indicating *no* relationship, when the number of same- and reverse-ordered pairs are *equal*. This situation is illustrated in Table 12.13.

The computation of gamma involves predicting whether there are more same- or more reverse-ordered pairs of observations. Following the PRE format, we will first make this prediction on the basis of knowledge about one variable only. We will then measure how much our predictive success is improved by basing predictions on information about the distribution of observations on both variables. The prediction rules and definitions of error for gamma are as follows.

Table 12.11. Pattern of Ordered Pairs for a Perfect Positive Relationship

	Variable Y		
Variable X	Low	Medium	High
Low	●		
Medium		●	
High			●

Table 12.12. Pattern of Ordered Pairs for a Perfect Negative Relationship

	Variable Y		
Variable X	Low	Medium	High
Low			●
Medium		●	
High	●		

Table 12.13. Pattern of Ordered Pairs for No Relationship

Variable X	Variable Y		
	Low	Medium	High
Low	●	●	●
Medium	●	●	●
High	●	●	●

Prediction Rule 1: For each ordered pair of observations, predict that it is either same- or reverse-ordered by *guessing*. Given information about the distribution of observations on one variable only, we have no information as to whether there are more same- or more reverse-ordered pairs. The chance that any given prediction made in this manner is correct is .5. In other words, we can expect to guess correctly half of the time and to guess incorrectly half of the time when given two possible choices. Therefore, surprising as it may seem, in the long run guessing will result in fewer prediction errors than any other prediction rule.

Errors Committed Using Rule 1 (E_1): The number of errors will equal one-half the total number of ordered pairs. Because the probability of making a correct prediction using rule 1 is .5, the probability of making a prediction error is equal to $1 - .5$, or .5.

Prediction Rule 2: For *each* ordered pair of observations, predict that it is same-ordered if the observed number of same-ordered pairs is larger than the observed number of reverse-ordered pairs; predict that it is reverse-ordered if the observed number of reverse-ordered pairs is larger than the observed number of same-ordered pairs.

Errors Committed Using Rule 2 (E_2): The number of errors will equal the observed number of same- or reverse-ordered pairs, whichever is *smaller*.

The conceptual formula for computing gamma is

$$\gamma = \frac{.5(n_s + n_r) - \min(n_s, n_r)}{.5(n_s + n_r)} \tag{12.3}$$

where γ = gamma

n_s = observed number of same-ordered pairs

n_r = observed number of reverse-ordered pairs

$\min(n_s, n_r)$ = *minimum* value available given n_s and n_r. In other words, the observed number of same- or reverse-ordered pairs, whichever is smaller

Note that the total number of observed *ordered* pairs is equal to $n_s + n_r$. Therefore $E_1 = .5(n_s + n_r)$, $E_2 = \min(n_s, n_r)$, and formula 12.3 follows the general PRE format:

$$\gamma = \frac{E_1 - E_2}{E_1}$$

Let us now compute a value of gamma for the relationship between preoperative stress level and postoperative recovery rate presented in Table 12.14. Visual examination of Table 12.14 shows that there is a negative relationship, with recovery rate tending to be above average (high) when stress is low and below average (low) when stress is high. In order to compute a value of gamma for this relationship it will first be necessary to convert the percentages into frequencies, as displayed in Table 12.15.

To find n_s multiply each cell frequency by the sum of the frequencies in all cells that are *below and to the right* of that cell, then sum the resulting products. For Table 12.15, beginning with the upper left-hand cell,

$$n_s = 3(31 + 17 + 16 + 6) + 19(17 + 6) + 16(16 + 6) + 31(6)$$
$$= 1,185$$

Table 12.14. Preoperative Stress Level and Postoperative Recovery Rate

	Stress level (%)		
Recovery rate	Low	Medium	High
Below average	5.0	28.8	66.2
Average	26.7	47.0	25.0
Above Average	68.3	24.2	8.8
Total	100.0	100.0	100.0
N	60	66	68

Table 12.15. Preoperative Stress Level and Postoperative Recovery Rate

	Stress level (frequency)		
Recovery rate	Low	Medium	High
Below average	3	19	45
Average	16	31	17
Above average	41	16	6
Total	60	66	68

To find n_r multiply each cell frequency by the sum of the frequencies in all cells that are *below and to the left* of that cell, then sum the resulting products. For Table 12.15, beginning with the upper right-hand cell,

$$n_r = 45(31 + 16 + 16 + 41) + 19(16 + 41)$$
$$+ 17(16 + 41) + 31 (41)$$
$$= 8,003$$

Because n_s is smaller than n_r in this example, the value $\min(n_s , n_r)$ is equal to n_s, or 1185.

According to formula 12.3, a value of gamma for Table 12.15 is computed as

$$\gamma = \frac{.5(n_s + n_r) - \min(n_s , n_r)}{.5(n_s + n_r)} = \frac{.5(1185 + 8003) - 1185}{.5(1185 + 8003)}$$

$$= \frac{.5(9188) - 1185}{.5(9188)} = \frac{4594 - 1185}{4594} = \frac{3409}{4594} = .74$$

However, because the relationship in Table 12.15 is negative, as indicated by a greater number of reverse-ordered than same-ordered pairs, a minus sign must be affixed to this value. Therefore the value of gamma for Table 12.15 is $-.74$.

The computation of gamma is simplified considerably by the use of formula 12.4, which not only involves fewer computations but also will automatically yield a negative value for a negative relationship.[4]

$$\gamma = \frac{n_s - n_r}{n_s + n_r} \tag{12.4}$$

For Table 12.15,

$$\gamma = \frac{n_s - n_r}{n_s + n_r} = \frac{1185 - 8003}{1185 + 8003} = \frac{-6818}{9188} = -.74$$

INTERPRETATION

The value $-.74$ obtained for Table 12.15 indicates a strong negative relationship between preoperative stress level and postoperative recovery rate. According to the PRE approach, 74 percent of the prediction errors initially committed by guessing whether each pair of observations was same- or reverse-ordered were reduced or eliminated when predictions were based on knowledge about the bivariate distribution of

[4] For the derivation of formula 12.4 from formula 12.3 see Mueller, Schuessler, and Costner (1977).

observations displayed in Table 12.15. Furthermore, because stress level is treated as the independent variable and recovery rate as the dependent variable in Table 12.14, it may also be concluded that preoperative stress level explains 74 percent of the variation in postoperative recovery rate.

It is important to note, however, that, because gamma is a symmetrical measure, exactly the same value, −.74, would apply if the independent and dependent variables were reversed (although it would not be logical to consider *post*operative recovery rate as having a causal influence upon *pre*operative stress level).

A disadvantage of gamma, which will be further discussed in the following sections, is that gamma may be misleading regarding the strength of a relationship because it does not consider all possible pairs of observations. As we have seen, the computation of gamma considers ordered pairs only, excluding pairs that are tied on either one or both variables. Whenever the number of observations (N) exceeds the number of ordered categories on either variable, as is almost always the case, some tied pairs are inevitable. The proportion of tied pairs, however, is usually not sufficiently large to have a significant effect on the computed value of gamma. But when the proportion of tied pairs is large, the computation of gamma is based on a small, and possibly negligible, proportion of all possible pairs. Also, while any given bivariate distribution of observations will yield only one value of gamma, the same value of gamma may be obtained for many alternative distributions. An excellent discussion of these and other disadvantages of gamma is presented by Mueller, Schuessler, and Costner (1970) and therefore will not be repeated here. Most of these problems may be avoided, however, by maximizing the potential number of untied, or ordered, pairs. This may generally be accomplished by arranging a data set so that each variable has as many ordered categories as is practicable, with nearly uniform marginal distributions.

SIGNIFICANCE

The statistical significance of a computed value of gamma may be tested by transforming it into a normal distribution value (z score) via formula 12.5:

$$z = \gamma \sqrt{\frac{n_s + n_r}{N(1 - \gamma^2)}} \tag{12.5}$$

The null hypothesis being tested here is that gamma does not significantly differ from zero ($H_0 : \gamma = 0$). Either a one- or a two-tailed region of rejection may be specified, and the level of significance is determined by referring the value computed according to formula 12.5 to Table C.2 in Appendix C.

For example, to test the significance of the value of gamma that was computed for Table 12.15,

$$z = \gamma \sqrt{\frac{n_s + n_r}{N(1 - \gamma^2)}} = -.74 \sqrt{\frac{1185 + 8003}{194[1 - (-.74)^2]}}$$

$$= -.74 \sqrt{\frac{9188}{194\,(.45)}} = -.74 \sqrt{\frac{9188}{87.3}} = -.74 \sqrt{105.25}$$

$$= -.74(10.26) = -7.59$$

For a one-tailed test ($H_1 : \gamma < 0$), a z score of -7.59 is significant beyond the .001 level. Therefore the inference decision is to reject the null hypothesis; the value of gamma computed for Table 12.15 is statistically significant.

2 X 2 TABLES AND YULE'S Q

Gamma may be computed for a cross-tabulation of *any* size. That is, a table may contain any number of rows and columns.[5] But Yule's Q is the ordinal measure of association that researchers have long used for data cast into a 2 X 2 table. When the cells of a 2 X 2 table are labeled according to the scheme presented in Table 12.16, Yule's Q is computed as

$$Q = \frac{ad - bc}{ad + bc} \tag{12.6}$$

This situation is simplified, however, when it is recognized that, because ad $= n_s$ and bc $= n_r$, Yule's Q is the equivalent of gamma when computed for a 2 X 2 table. That is,

$$Q = \frac{n_s - n_r}{n_s + n_r} = \gamma$$

Therefore Yule's Q test may be readily understood as simply a special case of gamma.

Table 12.16. Schematic Representation of Cells for Computation of Yule's Q

	Variable Y	
Variable X	A	B
A	a	b
B	c	d

[5] Although there is no upper limit, there is a minimum of two categories for each variable.

Another important aspect of gamma and 2 × 2 tables is that *gamma may be computed for any 2 × 2 table regardless of the level of measurement.* Gamma, an ordinal level measure of association, may be applied to the analysis of *nominal* level data in the special case of a 2 × 2 table. The explanation for this is that the dichotomized categories of any variable may be considered as opposite extremes of a continuum. Thus, even a variable such as patients' sex, recorded in the categories male and female, may be treated as ordinal level because the measurement may be considered as indicating whether an individual is more or less feminine, for example.[6] This approach to dichotomous nominal variables allows the researcher increased flexibility in the analysis and permits the use of a measure of association that will also indicate the nature of the relationship.

For example, a value of gamma may be computed thus for the relationship between smoking behavior and death due to lung cancer presented in Table 12.1:

$$\gamma = \frac{n_s - n_r}{n_s + n_r} = \frac{288 - 8}{288 + 8} = \frac{280}{296} = +.95$$

This result indicates a strong positive association, with the probability of death due to lung cancer increasing with the degree of smoking. On the other hand, the value of gamma for Table 12.2 is

$$\gamma = \frac{n_s - n_r}{n_s + n_r} = \frac{8 - 288}{8 + 288} = \frac{-280}{296} = -.95$$

indicating a strong negative association. This measure is much more useful than our previous attempts to examine these relationships by using chi-square and lambda.

Somers' *d*

Somers' *d* is an asymmetrical proportional reduction in error measure of association between two ordinal level variables. Its value may range from −1.00 to +1.00. As mentioned in the discussion of gamma, Somers' *d* is an extension of gamma and is similarly concerned with predicting the relative order of pairs of observations.

COMPUTATION

A general formula for the computation of Somers' *d* is presented in formula 12.7.

---

[6] In fact, researchers often e⸍tend this approach to treat dichotomous nominal variables as interval level measurements by assigning a value of 0 to one category and 1 to the other. This is called *dummy variable analysis* and is discussed in Loether and McTavish (1974a p. 333), and Blalock (1972, p. 498).

$$d = \frac{n_s - n_r}{n_s + n_r + T_d} \tag{12.7}$$

where d = Somer's d

n_s = observed number of same-ordered pairs

n_r = observed number of reverse-ordered pairs

T_d = observed number of pairs that are tied on the dependent variable but not on the independent variable

The numerator of formula 12.7 is identical to that of formula 12.4 for the computation of gamma. The denominator differs only in the addition of the expression T_d. T_d is added because Somers' d is a measure of the extent to which the ordering of pairs of observations may be successfully predicted for the dependent variable. Because no prediction of order will be successful for pairs of observations that are tied on the dependent variable, such tied pairs are treated as prediction errors in the computation of Somers' d. Pairs of observations that are tied on both variables are not included in formula 12.7 because predictions must be based on an observed order on the independent variable. It is not possible to make a rational prediction of order on the dependent variable for pairs that are tied on the independent variable. Thus, the denominator of formula 12.7 includes all the pairs for which a prediction of order on the dependent variable is possible.

When variable Y is designated as the dependent variable, Somers' d is computed as

$$d_{yx} = \frac{n_s - n_r}{n_s + n_r + T_y} \tag{12.8}$$

The subscript yx following d in formula 12.8 indicates that variable Y is being predicted from variable X, and T_y is the observed number of pairs that are tied on variable Y only. This notation is important because, as with lambda, a different value of Somers' d will be obtained if variable X is considered dependent upon variable Y. This latter value is computed according to formula 12.9

$$d_{xy} = \frac{n_s - n_r}{n_s + n_r + T_x} \tag{12.9}$$

in which d_{xy} indicates that variable X is being predicted from variable Y, and T_x is the observed number of pairs that are tied on variable X only.

As stated earlier in reference to Table 12.7, the number of pairs tied on variable Y but not on variable X are found by multiplying the frequency of each cell by the sum of all observations located within the same column or row of the table (depending on where the dependent variable is located) and then summing these products. Thus for Table 12.15, considering postoperative recovery rate as the dependent variable (Y), $T_y = 3(19 + 45) + 19(45) + 16(31 + 17) + 31(17) + 41(16 + 6) + 16(6) = 3,340$. In the previous computation of gamma it was found that $n_s = 1,185$ and $n_r = 8,003$. Therefore according to formula 12.8

$$d_{yx} = \frac{n_s - n_r}{n_s + n_r + T_y} = \frac{1185 - 8003}{1185 + 8003 + 3340} = \frac{-6818}{12,528}$$

$$= -.54$$

INTERPRETATION
The value $-.54$ indicates a moderate negative relationship between preoperative stress and postoperative recovery rate, with preoperative stress explaining 54 percent of the variation in postoperative recovery rate. This result is lower than that obtained for gamma for Table 12.15 ($\gamma = -.74$) because it includes *all* errors committed in predicting order on the dependent variable from the observed order on the independent variable.

SIGNIFICANCE
The statistical significance of a computed value of Somers' d may be tested by formula 12.10, which provides a test of the null hypothesis that Somers' d does not significantly differ from zero ($H_0 : d = 0$).

$$z = \frac{n_s - n_r}{\sqrt{\dfrac{N(N - 1)(2N + 5)}{18}}} \qquad (12.10)$$

Either a one- or two-tailed region of rejection may be specified. The level of significance is determined by reference to Table C.2.

To test the significance of the value of Somers' d that was computed for Table 12.15:

$$z = \frac{-6818}{\sqrt{\dfrac{(194)(193)[2(194) + 5]}{18}}} = \frac{-6818}{\sqrt{\dfrac{(194)(193)(393)}{18}}}$$

$$= \frac{-6818}{\sqrt{\dfrac{14,714,706}{18}}} = \frac{-6818}{\sqrt{817,483.67}} = \frac{-6818}{904.15} = -7.54$$

For a one-tailed test ($H_1 : d < 0$), a z score of -7.54 is significant beyond the .001 level. Therefore the inference decision is to reject the null hypothesis; the value of Somers' d computed for Table 12.15 is statistically significant.

Kendall's Tau

Also referred to as *Kendall's rank-order correlation coefficient*, Kendall's tau (τ) is a symmetrical proportional reduction in error measure of association between two ordinal level variables. Its value may range from -1.00 to $+1.00$.

Like gamma, Kendall's tau is a measure of how well the relative order of pairs of observations may be predicted. Kendall's tau is a more conservative measure of ordinal association than gamma, however, inasmuch as for any given set of observations the value of tau will generally be lower than that of gamma. Another way of viewing this difference is that Kendall's tau is a more demanding measure of association than gamma, because tau employs a more rigid definition of what constitutes perfect association. There are three forms of Kendall's tau, which will be discussed individually. In each case the numerator of the computational formula is identical to that for gamma and Somers' d (see formulas 12.4 and 12.7 respectively).

Tau_a

COMPUTATION

Kendall's tau_a is a measure of the relative preponderance of same- or reverse-ordered pairs *out of all possible unique pairs* of observations. Thus, as indicated in formula 12.11, the denominator of the computational formula for tau_a includes untied pairs, pairs tied on variable Y only, pairs tied on variable X only, and pairs tied on both variables X and Y.

$$\tau_a = \frac{n_s - n_r}{T} \tag{12.11}$$

where τ_a = Kendall's tau_a

$\quad n_s$ = observed number of same-ordered pairs

$\quad n_r$ = observed number of reverse-ordered pairs

$\quad T$ = number of all possible unique pairs, computed as $N(N-1)/2$

In contrast with gamma, which may reach a value of 1.00 even when there are many tied pairs, if any ties are present, as they usually are, tau_a cannot reach a value of 1.00. This is because the denominator of tau_a, which includes tied pairs, will be greater than either n_s or n_r. For this reason tau_a is not often used.

For Table 12.15 $n_s = 1185$, $n_r = 8003$ (see computation of gamma), and $T = \dfrac{N(N-1)}{2} = \dfrac{194(193)}{2} = 18{,}721$. According to formula 12.11, Kendall's tau_a is computed as

$$\tau_a = \frac{n_s - n_r}{T} = \frac{1185 - 8003}{18{,}721} = \frac{-6818}{18{,}721} = -.36$$

INTERPRETATION

The value $-.36$ indicates a mild negative relationship between preoperative stress and postoperative recovery rate, with 36 percent of the variation in either variable being explained by the other. This result is slightly lower than that obtained for Somers' d_{yx} ($d_{yx} = -.54$) and much lower than that obtained for gamma ($\gamma = -.74$) for Table 12.15.

SIGNIFICANCE

The statistical significance of a computed value of Kendall's tau_a may be tested by a transformation into the normal distribution according to formula 12.12.

$$z = \frac{\tau_a}{\sqrt{\dfrac{2(2N + 5)}{9N(N-1)}}} \tag{12.12}$$

The null hypothesis being tested is that tau_a does not significantly differ from zero ($H_0 : \tau_a = 0$). Either a one- or a two-tailed region of rejection may be specified, and the level of significance is determined by looking up the z value obtained in Table C.2.

To test the significance of the value of Kendall's tau_a that was computed for Table 12.15,

$$z = \frac{\tau_a}{\sqrt{\dfrac{2(2N + 5)}{9N(N- 1)}}} = \frac{-.36}{\sqrt{\dfrac{2[2(194) + 5]}{9(194)\,(193)}}} = \frac{-.36}{\sqrt{\dfrac{786}{336{,}978}}} = \frac{-.36}{\sqrt{.0023}}$$

$$= \frac{-.36}{.048} = -7.50$$

For a one-tailed test ($H_1 : \tau_a < 0$), a z score of -7.50 is significant beyond the .001 level. Therefore the inference decision is to reject the null hypothesis; the value of Kendall's tau_a computed for Table 12.15 is statistically significant.

Tau_b

COMPUTATION

In contrast with tau_a, the computational formula for tau_b (τ_b) excludes from the denominator any pairs that are tied on *both* variables. Such pairs may be considered trivial because the main focus of association is on the pattern of the distribution of observations in different cells of a table rather than the number of observations that are located within the same cell.

Kendall's tau$_b$ may be computed according to formula 12.13:

$$\tau_b = \frac{n_s - n_r}{\sqrt{(n_s + n_r + T_y)(n_s + n_r + T_x)}} \qquad (12.13)$$

where τ_b = Kendall's tau$_b$

n_s = observed number of same-ordered pairs

n_r = observed number of reverse-ordered pairs

T_y = observed number of pairs that are tied on variable Y only

T_x = observed number of pairs that are tied on variable X only

For Table 12.15, considering postoperative recovery rates as variable Y and preoperative stress as variable X,

$$T_y = 3(19 + 45) + 19(45) + 16(31 + 17) + 31(17)$$
$$+ 41(16 + 6) + 16(6)$$
$$= 3340$$

(as was previously computed for Somers' d_{yx}) and

$$T_x = 3(16 + 41) + 16(41) + 19(31 + 16) + 31(16)$$
$$+ 45(17 + 6) + 17(6)$$
$$= 3353$$

From previous computations we know that $n_s = 1185$ and $n_r = 8003$. Therefore, according to formula 12.13 the value of Kendall's tau$_b$ for Table 12.15 is computed as

$$\tau_b = \frac{n_s - n_r}{\sqrt{(n_s + n_r + T_y)(n_s + n_r + T_x)}}$$

$$= \frac{1185 - 8003}{\sqrt{(1185 + 8003 + 3340)(1185 + 8003 + 3353)}}$$

$$= \frac{-6818}{\sqrt{(12,528)(12,541)}} = \frac{-6818}{\sqrt{157,113,648}} = \frac{-6818}{12,534.5}$$

$$= -.54$$

INTERPRETATION

The value $-.54$ indicates a moderate negative relationship between preoperative stress and postoperative recovery rate, with 54 percent of the variation in either variable being explained by the other. Because pairs of observations that are tied on both variables are excluded from the denominator of formula 12.13, this value of tau_b is slightly higher than the value of tau_a ($\tau_a = -.36$) that was also computed for Table 12.15. This value of tau_b, however, is identical with that of Somers' d_{yx}, which was computed previously. Whenever T_y is equal (or approximately equal) to T_x, tau_b will be identical (or very similar) to Somers' d. But, for a given set of observations, if T_y is not equal to T_x, the computed value of tau_b will be smaller than that of Somers' d, because tau_b considers pairs that are tied on either variable. Therefore the denominator of formula 12.13 will be larger than that of formula 12.7 in such cases.

A disadvantage of tau_b is that it cannot reach a value of 1.00 if the table for which it is computed is not square, that is, if the number of rows and columns are not equal ($R \neq C$). An adjustment for tables that are not square is included in the computation of tau_c, which is presented in the following section.

SIGNIFICANCE

The statistical significance of a computed value of Kendall's tau_b may be tested by formula 12.10, which was introduced in the discussion of Somers' d. To understand why the same formula may be applied to test the significance of more than one measure, we must recall that Somers' d and Kendall's tau_b have identical numerators. Furthermore, rather than testing the value of d or tau_b directly, formula 12.10 actually provides a test of the likelihood of obtaining a value as large as or greater than the numerator, $n_s - n_r$, by chance. Thus, formula 12.10 could also be applied to test the significance of gamma, although formula 12.5 provides a convenient shortcut for dealing with gamma.[7]

When applied to tau_b, formula 12.10 tests the null hypothesis that tau_b does not significantly differ from zero (H_0: $\tau_b = 0$)[8] and is computed for Table 12.15 as follows:

---

[7] For a further discussion see Somers (1968, p. 811), Weiss (1968, p. 269), and Freeman (1965, p. 171).

[8] Technically this formula is appropriate when the number of tied pairs is relatively small. A complicated adjustment factor should be included when the number of ties is large (Blalock, 1960, p. 324, Hays, 1963, p. 654). However, the adjustment factor is ignored here for several reasons. First, formula 12.10 is easier to compute. Second, statisticians are notoriously in disagreement when it comes to specifying what is meant by terms such as "relatively small" and "relatively large," and this case is no exception. Third, formula 12.10 provides a conservative test of significance in that the z score obtained is smaller than that which would be obtained using the adjustment for ties and therefore reduces the risk of a type I error, although the risk of a type II error is correspondingly increased.

$$z = \frac{n_s - n_r}{\sqrt{\dfrac{N(N-1)(2N+5)}{18}}} = \frac{-6818}{\sqrt{\dfrac{(194)(193)[2(194)+5]}{18}}}$$

$$= -7.54$$

As was the case for Somers' d, for a one-tailed test (H_1 : $\tau_b < 0$), a z score of -7.54 is significant beyond the .001 level. Therefore the inference decision is to reject the null hypothesis; the value of Kendall's tau_b computed for Table 12.15 is statistically significant.

Tau$_c$
COMPUTATION

Conceptually, Kendall's tau$_c$ (τ_c) is identical to tau$_b$ in that it is a PRE measure of ordinal association that can be applied to pairs of observations that are tied on either but not both variables. The difference between these two measures is that the computation of tau$_c$ includes an adjustment so that a maximum value of 1.00 may be obtained for *any* table whether it is square or not. Tau$_c$ may be computed according to formula 12.14:

$$\tau_c = \frac{2m(n_s - n_r)}{N^2(m-1)} \qquad (12.14)$$

where τ_c = Kendall's tau$_c$

n_s = observed number of same-ordered pairs

n_r = observed number of reverse-ordered pairs

N = total number of observations

m = number of rows or columns, whichever is the smaller

For Table 12.15, since the numbers of rows and columns are equal, $m = 3$, and tau$_c$ is computed as

$$\tau_c = \frac{2(3)(1185-8003)}{194^2(3-1)} = \frac{6(-6818)}{37,636(2)} = \frac{-40,908}{75,272} = -.54$$

INTERPRETATION AND SIGNIFICANCE

The value $-.54$ for tau$_c$ is identical to that obtained for tau$_b$ for Table 12.15. This should not be surprising, because tau$_c$ is an extension of tau$_b$. Although the values of tau$_b$ and tau$_c$ will not always be identical, they will be very similar. Therefore the discussion of the interpretation and significance of Kendall's tau$_b$ in the previous section is also applicable to tau$_c$.

Tau$_c$ should be computed for nonsquare tables, because a

Table 12.17. Comparison of Measures of Ordinal Association Computed for Table 12.15

Measure	Computed value	z	p
Gamma	$\gamma = -.74$	-7.59	$< .001$
Somers' d	$d = -.54$	-7.54	$< .001$
Kendall's tau_a	$\tau_a = -.36$	-7.50	$< .001$
Kendall's tau_b	$\tau_b = -.54$	-7.54	$< .001$
Kendall's tau_c	$\tau_c = -.54$	-7.54	$< .001$

value of 1.00 cannot be obtained for tau_b regardless of the strength of the relationship displayed in such a table. Tau_b is preferred for analyzing square tables, however, because tau_c will tend to understate the strength of a relationship in a square table.

Comparing Measures of Ordinal Association

We have just discussed and computed five PRE measures of ordinal association for Table 12.15. The results of these separate analyses of a single set of data are summarized in Table 12.17 for comparison. Note that the computed value of gamma is the largest ($-.74$), followed by Somers' d, Kendall's tau_b, and tau_c ($-.54$), and that Kendall's tau_a ($-.36$) is the smallest. Although each of these measures was computed for a single set of data using a common logical approach (PRE), their values differ according to how tied pairs are handled in their computation.

Kendall's tau_b and tau_c are equal to Somers' d for Table 12.15, because T_y is approximately equal to T_x, as was noted in the discussion of tau_b. But when T_y is not equal to T_x, as is usually the case, the order of magnitude of these measures will typically be as follows: gamma will be the largest, followed by Somers' d, Kendall's tau_b, and Kendall's tau_c, with Kendall's tau_a having the smallest value. This order results from the fact that the computational formulas for these measures contain the same expression $(n_s - n_r)$ in their numerators but include increasingly more tied pairs in their denominators.[9] That is, while gamma includes no tied pairs, Somers' d includes pairs that are tied on the dependent variable only, Kendall's tau_b and tau_c include pairs that are tied on either variable but not both, and Kendall's tau_a includes all possible pairs.

Because each of these measures provides a unique analysis of any given data set, it is not appropriate to make comparisons

[9] In the very rare case in which there are *no* tied pairs, each of these measures will have exactly the same value.

between the size of their values. Thus, gamma should not be judged to be the "best" or "strongest" measure of association in this group because it yields the highest value. Its value is relatively high by virtue of the process involved in its computation, not because the relationship is any stronger when gamma is computed than when the other measures are. The data remain unchanged. This is further supported by the fact that each of the measures computed for Table 12.15 is significant beyond the .001 level, with similar z score values ranging from -7.50 to -7.59.

The decision regarding which of these measures should be used in any given case will depend upon two major criteria. First, if the main interest is in examining whether a causal relationship exists between two variables, an asymmetrical measure should be selected. The choice in that case would have to be Somers' d, because it is the only asymmetrical measure in the group. If the main interest lies in examining the degree to which variation on each of two variables tends to coincide without regard to the direction of causation, then a symmetrical measure should be selected.

Second, if it is decided that a symmetrical measure is needed, a choice must then be made between gamma and Kendall's tau. The main distinction between these measures is that gamma ignores tied pairs and is almost always computed on less than the entire data set, while Kendall's tau includes tied pairs, treating them as prediction errors. Thus the decision as to which measure to use depends to a large extent upon how one prefers to define tied pairs: that is, whether they are to be considered prediction errors or not. An additional consideration is that gamma is much easier to compute and test for statistical significance than Kendall's tau, and this probably accounts for the tendency for gamma to be encountered in the research literature more often. On the other hand, because the value of tau will almost always be smaller than gamma, tau may be regarded as a more conservative measure and will help guard against attributing greater strength to a relationship than the data actually warrant.

A good rule of thumb is to use gamma when there are relatively few tied pairs and Kendall's tau when the number of ties is relatively large. As mentioned in the discussion of gamma, the number of ties may be reduced by increasing the number of ordinal categories. As this is done, the size of the table increases, and the computational simplicity of gamma is an advantage. But when the number of ties is relatively large, as is usually the case for small tables, especially a 2 × 2 table, Kendall's tau is generally preferred because less data is lost by including tied pairs. Furthermore the computation of tau is less complex for small tables than it is for large ones.

Table 12.18. Incidence of Birth Abnormalities by Maternal Stress

Birth condition	Maternal stress level	
	Not stressed	Stressed
Without abnormality	89 (100%)	92 (95%)
With abnormality	0 (0%)	5 (5%)
Total	89 (100%)	97 (100%)

To demonstrate the degree to which one may be misled by gamma when the number of ties is relatively large, let us consider Table 12.18. Examination of the percentage distributions reveals almost no relationship between maternal stress and the likelihood of a birth abnormality, with a large majority of both nonstressed and stressed mothers delivering infants without an abnormality. However, computing gamma for Table 12.18 we obtain the following result:

$$\gamma = \frac{n_s - n_r}{n_s + n_r} = \frac{445 - 0}{445 + 0} = \frac{445}{445} = +1.00$$

In contrast to the percentage distributions, this value indicates an extremely strong relationship; in fact, it indicates a "perfect" association between maternal stress and birth condition. On the other hand, computing Kendall's tau$_b$ we obtain

$$
\begin{aligned}
\tau_b &= \frac{n_s - n_r}{\sqrt{(n_s + n_r + T_y)(n_s + n_r + T_x)}} \\
&= \frac{445 - 0}{\sqrt{(445 + 0 + 8188)(445 + 0 + 460)}} = \frac{445}{\sqrt{(8633)(905)}} \\
&= \frac{445}{\sqrt{7,812,865}} = \frac{445}{2795.15} = +.16
\end{aligned}
$$

This value of tau indicates a very weak relationship between maternal stress and birth condition and is much more in accord with the analysis of the percentage distribution displayed in Table 12.18. This analysis of Table 12.18 demonstrates a major disadvantage of gamma, which is that its value will equal ± 1.00 whenever *any* cell in a 2 $\times$ 2 table is equal to 0, regardless of the number of observations located in the remaining cells.

WORKING WITH AND INTERPRETING DATA

1. For the following table, select the most appropriate measure of association and justify your choice. Then compute its value and interpret the result.

Table 1. Incidence of Thromboembolism Among Women Taking Oral Contraceptives, According to Blood Group

Blood group	Thromboembolism		Total
	Yes	No	
A	32	51	83
B	8	19	27
AB	6	5	11
O	9	70	79
Total	55	145	200

2. Compute and compare the values of gamma, Somers' d, and Kendall's tau to measure the association between blood pressure levels of a group of 92 fathers and their first-born children as displayed in Table 2. Remember to test the computed values for statistical significance. Interpret your results.

Table 2. Blood Pressure Level of Father and of First-Born Child at Age 15

Father's B.P.	Child's B.P.		
	Low	Normal	High
Low	15	8	5
Normal	9	11	11
High	3	7	23

3. Compute the value of Kendall's tau for the following table and test it for significance. Interpret your results.

Table 3. Percent RDA Caloric Intake by Age

Percent RDA caloric intake	Age		
	20–45	46–65	Over 65
0–25	0	3	4
26–50	3	7	1
51–75	8	2	0
76–100	10	1	0

4. The authors of the following articles analyze relationships between two variables. For each article, describe and interpret the findings and evaluate the appropriateness of the author's use of measures of association.

231

Denton, John A., and Vance B. Wisenbaker, Jr. Death experience and death anxiety among nurses and nursing students. *Nursing Research* 26:61–64, 1977. See Table 2.

Woods, Nancy Fugate, and Jo Anne L. Earp. Women with cured breast cancer: a study of mastectomy patients in North Carolina. *Nursing Research* 27:279–285, 1978. See Table 3.

5. The authors of the following articles present cross-classification tables but do not report measures of association. Select and compute an appropriate measure of association for the tables indicated below. Does your result support the author's interpretation of these data?

Downs, Florence S. Maternal stress in primigravidas as a factor in the production of neonatal pathology. *Nursing Science* 2:348–367, 1964. See Table 2.

Kayser, Jeanie Schmit, and Fred A. Minnigerode. Increasing nursing students' interest in working with aged patients. *Nursing Research* 24:23–26, 1975. See Table 2.

Smith, Mary Colette. Patient responses to being transferred during hospitalization. *Nursing Research* 25: 192–196, 1976. See Table 2.

The preceding chapter discussed methods for examining the nature and degree of relationship between nominal and ordinal level variables. As a group, those methods are referred to as *measures of association.* By convention, measures that describe relationships between interval level variables are generally referred to as *measures of correlation*, or *correlation coefficients.* But the difference between measures of association and measures of correlation is largely one of semantics, because conceptually their purpose is identical: to describe the nature and strength of a relationship between variables. Furthermore this semantic distinction is not applied by statisticians in an absolute manner. For example, Kendall's tau, which was presented in Chapter 12 as a measure of association between ordinal variables, is also commonly referred to as Kendall's rank order correlation coefficient. Thus the terms *association* and *correlation* may be and are used interchangeably. Therefore the basic concept and purpose for the measures discussed in this chapter are the same as in Chapter 12. The main difference is in their computation.

Three measures of correlation will be mentioned in this chapter: (1) Pearson's product moment correlation coefficient, which is by far the most often used measure of correlation and is discussed at length here, is designed for use with interval level variables whose relationship is linear, tending to follow the pattern of a straight line when graphed. (2) The correlation ratio is used with interval level variables whose relationship is curvilinear, tending to follow the pattern of a curved line. (3) Spearman's rank order correlation coefficient is used with ordinal level variables in a manner similar to Kendall's tau. The computation and interpretation of all three of these measures follows the familiar proportional reduction in error (PRE) conceptual approach.

Linear regression is the specific procedure employed for making predictions of the value of an interval variable in the computation of Pearson's coefficient. But unlike the method of counting the number of ordered and/or tied pairs of observations that was used to compute gamma, Somers' *d*, and Kendall's tau, regression is a valuable analytic technique in its own right. Therefore most of this chapter will be an extensive discussion of this method, which is followed by a discussion of Pearson's correlation coefficient and a note on other correlation methods.

Linear Regression

Data Requirements

The minimum requirements of the data if a linear regression (and correlation) analysis is to be performed are an interval level of measurement and an equal number of observations in each data set. That is, a linear regression and correlation analysis may be performed in either of two situations. One is when a single variable has been measured at the interval level for two groups containing an equal number of observations. For example, in an investigation to explore whether hypertension is hereditary, one might examine the relationship between fathers' and sons' blood pressure readings for 200 father-son pairs. Thus there would be a total of 200 bivariate observations consisting of a blood pressure reading for each father and his son. The other situation is when measurements have been obtained on each of two interval variables for one group of subjects. For example, in a dietary study the relationship between body weight and percent RDA (recommended daily allowance) caloric intake might be examined for a group of 75 patients, in which case there would be a total of 75 bivariate observations consisting of a body weight and percent RDA caloric intake measurement for each patient.

In the preceding chapter, measures of association were developed for nominal and ordinal level variables by predicting either a particular category or a particular order on one variable on the basis of an observed category or order on another variable. Prediction errors were measured by simply counting the number of times a wrong prediction was made. But when dealing with interval level variables, specific values of one variable may be predicted on the basis of values observed on another variable, and prediction errors may be measured more precisely by examining the number of measurement units by which the predicted values differ from the values actually observed. Regression is a method for predicting values on one interval variable from values observed on another.

Scatter Diagrams

The first step in performing a linear regression analysis is to plot a graph, called a *scatter diagram*, of all the bivariate interval level observations. In a scatter diagram (see Figure 13.1), one set of interval level observations are located along the horizontal axis, which is marked off from low to high from left to right, and the other set of interval level observations are located along the vertical axis, which is marked off from low to high from bottom to top.

It is important to examine a scatter diagram of a data set prior to performing a linear regression analysis in order to determine whether the data are arranged in a pattern that is approximately *linear*. As the name implies, linear regression is designed to analyze relationships that tend to follow a straight-line pattern. That is, the computations involved in performing a linear regression assume that the variables change (either increase or decrease) at a relatively fixed or constant rate. The final step in a linear regression analysis is the drawing, referred to as *fitting* by statisticians, of a straight line through the set of data points. This straight line, or *regression line*, represents or summarizes the trend displayed by the data. It may be thought of as indicating the central tendency of the set of bivariate observations.

It is not essential that all the points be arranged perfectly along a straight line, a situation which is extremely rare in actual practice. It is sufficient that they display a pattern that approximates, or suggests, a linear pattern. For our purposes it will be sufficient to determine visually whether a data set displays a linear pattern. Although there are statistical methods of testing a data set for linearity, they are beyond the scope of this text.

Three basic patterns may be observed in a scatter diagram: random scatter, linear pattern, and curvilinear pattern. As displayed in diagram A, Figure 13.1, when the data points are scattered about in a random or haphazard fashion, no pattern is discernible, and it is not possible to predict in a systematic manner values of one variable on the basis of observed values of another. That is, it is not possible to draw a single straight line that will represent the entire data set. In fact, there are many straight lines that might be drawn through these points, each of which is equally useless because there is no apparent trend and no relationship. Thus it would not be useful to apply a regression analysis in such a situation.

Diagrams B–G of Figure 13.1 display linear patterns for which a linear regression analysis would be appropriate. The relationships in diagrams B–D are *positive*, because as one variable increases in value, so does the other. On the other hand, diagrams E–G display *negative* relationships, in which one variable decreases as values for the other variable increase. In the rare situation in which all the data points are arranged perfectly along a straight line, there are no prediction errors and the relationship is of maximum strength. As the arrangement of points departs from a perfect straight line, prediction errors are committed and the strength of the relationship is less than maximum. When the points lie within a relatively narrow lane about an imaginary straight line, as in diagrams B and E, relatively few prediction errors are committed and the relationship is strong. As the points become more widely scattered about the imaginary line, as in diagrams C, D, F, and G, more prediction errors are committed, indicating a weaker relationship.

Although the patterns in diagrams H and I display distinct relationships, they do not conform to a straight line, and therefore a linear regression analysis is not appropriate.

Random scatter

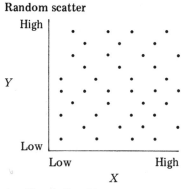

A. No relationship

Positive linear patterns

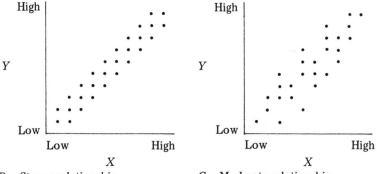

B. Strong relationship   C. Moderate relationship

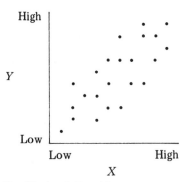

D. Weak relationship

Figure 13.1. Scatter diagram patterns.

Because of their curved shapes, patterns of this type are collectively referred to as *curvilinear*. Although there are many
possible curvilinear patterns, those displayed in diagrams H
and I are among the most common. For example, the U-
shaped pattern in diagram H would describe the relationship
between age (*X*) and number of physician visits during a
year (*Y*). The number of visits is typically high for children,

Negative linear patterns

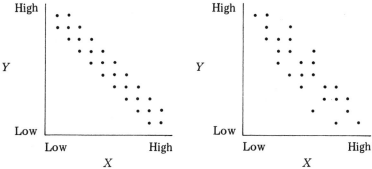

E. Strong relationship   F. Moderate relationship

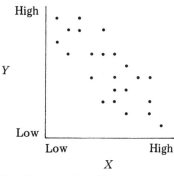

G. Weak relationship

Curvilinear patterns

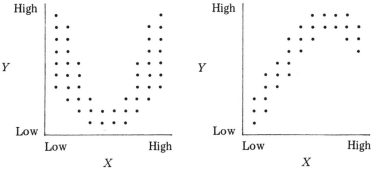

H. U-shaped relationship   I. J-shaped relationship

low for middle-aged adults, and high for the elderly. The pattern in diagram I would describe the relationship between age (X) and body weight (Y), with body weight increasing rapidly during childhood, slowing as adulthood is entered, leveling off during the middle adult ages, and then decreasing somewhat in old age.

Another reason for examining a scatter diagram is to

determine whether the data points conform to a single pattern. This aspect of a scatter diagram, referred to as *scedasticity*, indicates whether predictions of values for one variable can be made consistently on the basis of all values observed for the other variable. That is important because linear regression is based on a mathematical model that requires that values be predictable according to a uniform procedure for all observed values. It is appropriate to apply a linear regression analysis only to a data set that is *homoscedastic*, meaning that the data points are distributed uniformly throughout the pattern. Diagrams B through G of Figure 13.1 are examples of homoscedastic linear scatter patterns because the points conform to a single pattern, a straight line, in each case. Note that the strength of the relationship has no effect upon scedasticity. Also, although the curvilinear patterns displayed in diagrams H and I are homoscedastic, a linear regression analysis is not appropriate for them because they do not conform to a linear pattern.

Figure 13.2 displays a *heteroscedastic* data set, or one that does not conform to a single pattern. Although a linear pattern is apparent for the medium and high values of variable X, there is no pattern for the low values. Fitting a straight line to such a data set would not be appropriate, because the straight line would not be a good representative of the data points at low values of X. A pattern such as that displayed in Figure 13.2 might be observed for the relationship between income (X) and number of physician visits (Y) for a population in which the number of visits is low among low income persons who do not have access to or utilize programs such as Medicare and Medicaid but high among those who do, increasing in a positive linear fashion for the middle and high income groups.

Thus a linear regression analysis is appropriate for a set of bivariate interval level observations when the scatter diagram reveals a homoscedastic linear pattern. The scatter diagram also indicates whether a relationship is positive or negative and may suggest as well whether the relationship is strong,

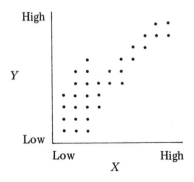

Figure 13.2. A heteroscedastic scatter pattern.

moderate, or weak. The measurement of the strength of the relationship will be discussed thoroughly in the section of this chapter that deals with Pearson's correlation coefficient.

Determining the "Best" Line

Upon visual examination of a scatter diagram that displays a linear relationship it is usually possible to draw a freehand trend line passing approximately through the center of the data points. But the problem with a freehand trend line is that each observer can draw a slightly different line to describe a single data set. For example, each of two observers has drawn a different trend line to describe the relationship between birth weight and gestational age displayed in Figure 13.3, and both lines appear to do equally well in that regard. Furthermore there is an infinite number of similar but different other lines that might be drawn through these points. The dilemma then is to decide which line is "best."

The main purpose of regression analysis is to predict, with the least amount of error, values of one variable on the basis of values observed on another. Because the regression line represents all possible predicted values, prediction error may be measured as the difference between the value actually observed for the predicted variable and the predicted value on the regression line. For example, using line A in Figure 13.3,

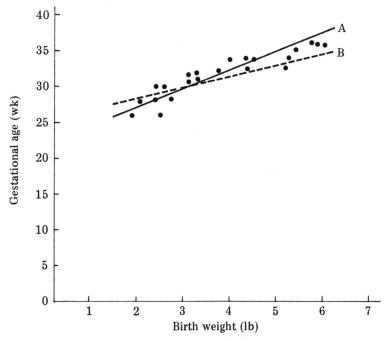

Figure 13.3. Scatter diagram of birth weight and gestational age for 22 infants with two freehand trend lines.

we may predict the gestational age of an infant whose birth weight is 4.2 pounds. We first locate 4.2 along the horizontal axis and then move vertically and perpendicularly from that point until we touch line A. We then read the predicted age value by moving to the left, parallel with the horizontal axis, until we touch the vertical axis. At that point the predicted value reads 32.5 weeks. But, as indicated in Table 13.1, the observed gestational age value for an infant whose birth weight is 4.2 pounds is 34 weeks, which yields a difference score of $+1.5$ $(34-32.5)$. Thus the observed value is 1.5 weeks higher than the predicted value. Similarly, the gestational age of an infant whose birth weight is 5.2 pounds would be predicted from line A as 35 weeks. As the observed value for 5.2 pounds is 33 weeks, the difference score is -2.0, indicating that the observed value is 2 weeks lower than the predicted value. The corresponding predicted values using line B are 32 (difference score, $+2.0$) and 33.5 (difference score, -0.5), respectively. If we were to continue in this manner, we could sum the difference scores for all predicted values, for each line; and the line with the smaller sum, either positive or negative, would be the better line, because the

Table 13.1. Birth Weight and Gestational Age for 22 Infants

Birth weight (lb)	Gestational age (wk)
1.9	26
2.1	28
2.5	28
2.5	30
2.6	30
2.6	26
2.8	28
3.1	32
3.1	31
3.3	32
3.3	31
3.8	32
4.2	34
4.6	34
4.6	33
4.8	34
5.2	33
5.3	34
5.5	35
5.8	36
5.9	36
6.2	36

smaller the sum of the difference scores, the less prediction error.

To find the best of all possible lines, then, one approach might be to repeat the above procedure for all lines possible and then select the one with the smallest prediction error. But since there are an infinite number of possible lines to be considered, this approach is not practical.

A standardized procedure has been formulated for determining the best-fitting line for a regression analysis. This line is located so as to make the sum of the difference scores (prediction errors) equal to zero. Thus the regression line is directly analogous to the mean of a univariate distribution, because the sum of deviations about the mean also sum to zero, and the regression line may be thought of as the mean of the bivariate data points. Also, like the mean of a univariate distribution, the sum of the squared deviations (difference scores) about the regression line is less than the sum of the squared deviations about any other line that might be considered. Therefore the regression line conforms to the least-squares principle introduced in Chapter 6 and is thus referred to as the *least-squares regression line*.

Fitting a Least-Squares Regression Line
COMPUTATIONAL PROCESS
A least-squares regression line is determined by plotting three predicted values, which are then connected by a straight line on a scatter diagram. The formula for a predicted value is

$$\hat{Y} = a_{yx} + b_{yx} X \qquad (13.1)$$

where $\hat{Y}$ = a predicted value of the dependent variable, Y

$\qquad a_{yx}$ = the Y-intercept

$\qquad b_{yx}$ = the slope

$\qquad X$ = an observed value of the independent variable, X

The symbol $\hat{Y}$ is read "Y-hat." All possible values of $Y(\hat{Y})$ are located on the regression line. The *Y-intercept* (a_{yx}) is the point at which the regression line crosses the vertical axis (note that the value of X will be zero at that point). The regression line does not necessarily pass through the origin of a scatter diagram; therefore, a_{yx} is usually not equal to zero. The *slope* (b_{yx}) indicates the predicted amount of change in variable Y that corresponds to a change of one unit in variable X.[1] For example, if b_{yx} = 2, then whenever

---

[1] The subscript $_{yx}$ used with the Y-intercept and slope indicates that they are computed for the regression of variable Y on variable X. That is, values of variable Y are being predicted from those observed for variable X. This distinction is important because different results will be obtained for the regression of variable X on variable Y. This will be discussed further later in this chapter.

the value of variable X increases by 1 unit on its measurement scale, variable Y will be expected to increase by 2 units on its measurement scale. The slope may also be negative, as in the case of a negative relationship. For example, if $b_{yx} = -1.5$, then variable Y will be expected to *decrease* by 1.5 units whenever variable X increases by 1 unit.

The formula for computing the value of the slope is

$$b_{yx} = \frac{N(\Sigma XY) - (\Sigma X)(\Sigma Y)}{N(\Sigma X^2) - (\Sigma X)^2} \tag{13.2}$$

Although formula 13.2 may appear quite formidable at first, the computation of the slope is largely a process of substituting readily available numbers for the symbols and performing the necessary arithmetic. In most cases the mean and standard deviation for the distributions of variables X and Y are computed to summarize the distributions before a regression analysis is attempted. From those computations the following values are already available: N, ΣX, ΣY, and ΣX^2. This leaves only ΣXY to be computed before proceeding to solve formula 13.2 for the value of b_{yx}.

After the slope has been obtained, the Y-intercept is computed as

$$a_{yx} = \overline{Y} - b_{yx}\overline{X} \tag{13.3}$$

All the values required to compute a_{yx} should be readily available to substitute in formula 13.3.[2]

A SIMPLE EXAMPLE
Before proceeding to fit a least-squares regression line to the birth weight and gestational age data, we will examine a very simple example to demonstrate how the process works. Figure 13.4 presents a scatter diagram for the relationship between the age of siblings for six pairs of siblings. The scatter diagram displays a homoscedastic positive linear pattern. In fact, the relationship appears to be perfect, and all the data points are expected to lie on the regression line. This is obviously a contrived example that is very unlikely to occur in actual practice.

The computations necessary for fitting the regression line are presented in Table 13.2. The slope (b_{yx}) has a value of $+2.0$, indicating that the relationship is positive and that variable Y (the age of the older sibling) will be expected to increase by two years for every one-year increase observed in variable X (the age of the younger sibling). This is easily verified by examining the X and Y columns of Table 13.2. When X increases

[2] An alternative formula is $a_{yx} = \dfrac{\Sigma Y - b_{yx}\,\Sigma X}{N}$

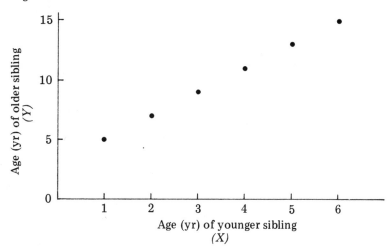

Figure 13.4. Scatter diagram of ages of six pairs of siblings.

Table 13.2. Computation of Regression Line for Ages of Six Pairs of Siblings

X	Y	XY	X^2
1	5	5	1
2	7	14	4
3	9	27	9
4	11	44	16
5	13	65	25
6	15	90	36
$\Sigma X = 21$	$\Sigma Y = 60$	$\Sigma XY = 245$	$\Sigma X^2 = 91$

$$\bar{X} = \frac{21}{6} = 3.5 \qquad \bar{Y} = \frac{60}{6} = 10$$

$$\bar{X} = \tfrac{\Sigma x / n}{}$$
$$\bar{y} = \tfrac{\Sigma y / n}{}$$

$$b_{yx} = \frac{N(\Sigma XY) - (\Sigma X)(\Sigma Y)}{N(\Sigma X^2) - (\Sigma X)^2} = \frac{6(245) - (21)(60)}{6(91) - 21^2} = \frac{1470 - 1260}{546 - 441}$$

$$= \frac{210}{105} = 2$$

$$a_{yx} = \bar{Y} - b_{yx}\bar{X} = 10 - 2(3.5) = 10 - 7 = 3$$

$$\hat{Y} = a_{yx} + b_{yx}X = 3 + 2X$$

from a value of 1 to 2, Y increases by two years from 5 to 7, and so on. The Y-intercept (a_{yx}) indicates that the regression line will cross the vertical axis where Y is equal to 3. The formula for predicting values of Y are generating the regression line is $\hat{Y} = 3 + 2X$.

As was mentioned earlier, three predicted values of Y are

needed to draw the regression line. Although it is true that any two points determine a straight line, it is advisable to plot a third value as a check for a possible error in computing the first two. Because the Y-intercept, by definition, lies on the regression line, the value of a_{yx} may be used as one of the points that determine the regression line. To repeat, a_{yx} is the value of Y when $X =$ zero. That is, when $X = 0$, $b_{yx} X = b_{yx} 0 = 0$, and $\hat{Y} = a_{yx} + 0 = a_{yx}$; or in the present case, $\hat{Y} = 3 + 2\,(0) = 3 + 0 = 3$. Because we now have a predicted Y value when X is low, let us now compute the $\hat{Y}$ value for a medium and a high value of X. Thus, when $X = 3$, $\hat{Y} = 3 + 2\,(3) = 3 + 6 = 9$; when $X = 6$, $\hat{Y} = 3 + 2\,(6) = 3 + 12 = 15$. The following points are then located on the scatter diagram and connected by a straight line, as in Figure 13.5: $X = 0$, $Y = 3$; $X = 3$, $Y = 9$; $X = 6$, $Y = 15$. The regression line should be labeled by writing the formula used to derive it, so that the reader may compute the predicted value of Y for any value of X that may be of interest. As was expected, all the data points lie on the regression line in Figure 13.5, indicating a perfect relationship; no prediction errors will be committed in predicting values of Y based on those observed for X in this case. That is, when the regression formula is used for this set of data, the predicted value of Y will be exactly equal to the observed value.

BIRTH WEIGHT AND GESTATIONAL AGE

Returning to the regression analysis of the relationship between birth weight and gestational age, the computations for plotting a least-squares regression line to predict gestational age from birth weight are presented in Table 13.3. In this case the slope is equal to 2.1, the Y-intercept has a value of 23.6, and the regression formula is $\hat{Y} = 23.6 + 2.1X$. To draw the regression line, the first point is plotted at the Y-intercept; that is, when $X = 0$, $\hat{Y} = 23.6$. Two additional

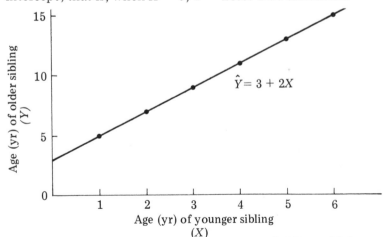

Figure 13.5. Scatter diagram of ages of six pairs of siblings with least-squares regression line.

Table 13.3. Computations for Regression of Gestational Age on Birth Weight

Birth weight (lb) X	Gestational age (wk) Y	XY	X^2
1.9	26	49.4	3.6
2.1	28	58.8	4.4
2.5	28	70.0	6.2
2.5	30	75.0	6.2
2.6	30	78.0	6.8
2.6	26	67.6	6.8
2.8	28	78.4	7.8
3.1	32	99.2	9.6
3.1	31	96.1	9.6
3.3	32	105.6	10.9
3.3	31	102.3	10.9
3.8	32	121.6	14.4
4.2	34	142.8	17.6
4.6	34	156.4	21.2
4.6	33	151.8	21.2
4.8	34	163.2	23.0
5.2	33	171.6	27.0
5.3	34	180.2	28.1
5.5	35	192.5	30.2
5.8	36	208.8	33.6
5.9	36	212.4	34.8
6.2	36	223.2	38.4
85.7	699	2804.9	372.3

$$\overline{X} = \frac{85.7}{22} = 3.9 \qquad \overline{Y} = \frac{699}{22} = 31.8$$

$$b_{yx} = \frac{N(\Sigma XY) - (\Sigma X)(\Sigma Y)}{N(\Sigma X^2) - (\Sigma X)^2} = \frac{22(2804.9) - (85.7)(699)}{22(372.3) - 85.7^2}$$

$$= \frac{61,707.8 - 59,904.3}{8,190.6 - 7,344.5} = \frac{1,803.5}{846.1} = 2.1$$

$$a_{yx} = \overline{Y} - b_{yx}\overline{X} = 31.8 - (2.1)(3.9) = 31.8 - 8.2 = 23.6$$

$$\hat{Y} = a_{yx} + b_{yx}X = 23.6 + 2.1X$$

points may be plotted by solving the regression equation for a value of $\hat{Y}$ when $X = 3$ and when $X = 6$, as follows: $\hat{Y} = 23.6 + (2.1)(3) = 29.9$, and $\hat{Y} = 23.6 + (2.1)(6) = 36.2$. We may thus plot points where $X = 3$, $Y = 29.9$ and where $X = 6$, $Y = 36.2$. Note that these points are plotted using xs to distinguish them from the solid dots that represent actual

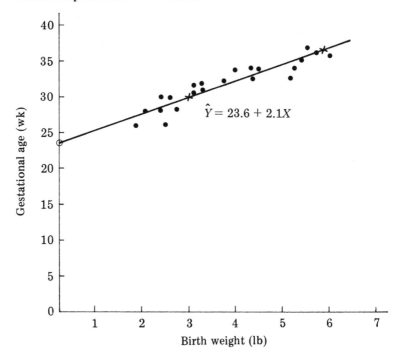

Figure 13.6. Scatter diagram of birth weight and gestational age with least-squares regression line for regression of gestational age on birth weight.

observations. The regression line is then drawn by connecting these points, as displayed in Figure 13.6.

As was mentioned earlier, the least-squares regression line may be considered as representing the mean of the bivariate observations on two variables, X and Y. Rather than present an in-depth discussion of the theoretical underpinnings of why this is so, we offer a brief demonstration in support of this statement. That is, if the least-squares regression line represents a mean, and if it is a good predictor of values for variable Y, the mean of the predicted values ($\hat{\bar{Y}}$) should be equal to the mean of the observed values ($\bar{Y}$). This may be verified by computing the predicted value of Y for each observed value of X and then computing the mean of the predicted values, as presented in Table 13.4. The mean in this case is 31.8, which is equal to the value computed for the mean of the observed Y values as presented in Table 13.3.

USE OF THE REGRESSION LINE

A basic use of the least-squares regression line is to describe the relationship between two variables. That is, a regression line that ascends from left to right, as in Figure 13.6, indicates a positive relationship, while a regression line that descends from left to right indicates a negative relationship.

The most important use of the least-squares regression line, however, is to predict values on one variable from values that

Table 13.4. Comparison of Mean of Predicted Values with Mean
of Observed Values

X	$\hat{Y} = 23.6 + 2.1X$
1.9	27.6
2.1	28.0
2.5	28.8
2.5	28.8
2.6	29.1
2.6	29.1
2.8	29.5
3.1	30.1
3.1	30.1
3.3	30.5
3.3	30.5
3.8	31.6
4.2	32.4
4.6	33.3
4.6	33.3
4.8	33.7
5.2	34.5
5.3	34.7
5.5	35.2
5.8	35.8
5.9	36.0
6.2	36.6
	699.2

$$\overline{\hat{Y}} = \frac{699.2}{22} = 31.8 = \overline{Y}$$

are observed on another variable. Thus, if an infant's birth
weight is known, gestational age may be conveniently predicted by referring to Figure 13.6. For example, the gestational age of an infant whose birth weight is 5 pounds may
be predicted by locating 5 along the horizontal axis and
moving perpendicularly from that point until the regression
line is reached. Then, by moving parallel to the horizontal
axis over to the vertical axis, the predicted gestational age
can be read as approximately 34 weeks. Alternatively, if a
more precise prediction is desired, the infant's gestational
age may be predicted by using the regression formula $\hat{Y} = 23.6$
$+ 2.1X$. Substituting the infant's birth weight of 5 pounds
for X we obtain: $\hat{Y} = 23.6 + (2.1)(5) = 34.1$.

It is important to note that the birth weight value (X) of
5 in this example is not one of those actually observed for
the group of 22 infants from which the regression formula
was computed. We make the assumption that data from infants other than the 22 who were observed will conform to

the positive linear trend observed in Figure 13.6, and we predict the gestational age of those infants by using the least-squares regression line and regression formula presented in Figure 13.6. It is appropriate to make predictions for such unobserved values, however, only when the given value of X is within the range of observed values from which the regression formula was computed. Thus the regression line presented in Figure 13.6 should be used to predict gestational age only for infants whose birth weight is between 1.9 and 6.2 pounds. This is because we have evidence, as presented in Figure 13.6, that there is a positive linear relationship between birth weight and gestational age for values within that range. We do not know whether the linear relationship will continue for birth weight values larger than 6.2. It is possible that the relationship may not exist, or may level off, once birth weight reaches a certain point, or that the relationship will become curvilinear.

PREDICTING BIRTH WEIGHT FROM GESTATIONAL AGE

The least-squares regression formula and line that were just computed in Table 13.3 and Figure 13.6 may be applied only in predicting gestational age from birth weight. They may *not* be applied in the reverse manner to predict birth weight from gestational age. For the latter purpose a separate regression analysis must be performed, which will yield a different regression formula and line.

For the analysis of the regression of birth weight on gestational age, the same basic computational procedures and formulas are used as for finding the regression of gestational age on birth weight. However, wherever an X appears in a formula, a Y will be substituted, and wherever a Y appears, an X will be substituted. Thus the slope is indicated as b_{xy} (indicating the regression of variable X on variable Y) and is computed by the following formula:

$$b_{xy} = \frac{N(\Sigma XY) - (\Sigma X)(\Sigma Y)}{N(\Sigma Y^2) - (\Sigma Y)^2} \tag{13.4}$$

This formula has the same numerator as formula 13.2 (for computing b_{yx}) but a different denominator. The *X-intercept*, the point at which the regression line will intersect the *X-axis* of the scatter diagram, is indicated as a_{xy} and is computed as

$$a_{xy} = \overline{X} - b_{xy}\overline{Y} \tag{13.5}$$

Finally, the regression formula for predicting values for variable X is

$$\hat{X} = a_{xy} + b_{xy}Y \tag{13.6}$$

These computations for the regression of birth weight on gestational age are presented in Table 13.5. The results for the slope, intercept, and regression formula should be compared with those presented in Table 13.3 to verify that they are different. In the case at hand, the slope has a value of .4, indicating that whenever gestational age increases by one week,

Table 13.5. Computations for Regression of Birth Weight on Gestational Age

Birth weight (lb) X	Gestational age (wk) Y	XY	Y^2
1.9	26	49.4	676
2.1	28	58.8	784
2.5	28	70.0	784
2.5	30	75.0	900
2.6	30	78.0	900
2.6	26	67.6	676
2.8	28	78.4	784
3.1	32	99.2	1024
3.1	31	96.1	961
3.3	32	105.6	1024
3.3	31	102.3	961
3.8	32	121.6	1024
4.2	34	142.8	1156
4.6	34	156.4	1156
4.6	33	151.8	1089
4.8	34	163.2	1156
5.2	33	171.6	1089
5.3	34	180.2	1156
5.5	35	192.5	1225
5.8	36	208.8	1296
5.9	36	212.4	1296
6.2	36	223.2	1296
85.7	699	2804.9	22,413

$$\overline{X} = \frac{85.7}{22} = 3.9 \qquad \overline{Y} = \frac{699}{22} = 31.8$$

$$b_{xy} = \frac{N(\Sigma XY) - (\Sigma X)(\Sigma Y)}{N(\Sigma Y^2) - (\Sigma Y)^2} = \frac{22(2804.9) - (85.7)(699)}{22(22,413) - 699^2}$$

$$= \frac{61,707.8 - 59,904.3}{493,086 - 488,601} = \frac{1,803.5}{4,485} = .4$$

$$a_{xy} = \overline{X} - b_{xy}\overline{Y} = 3.9 - (.4)(31.8) = 3.9 - 12.7 = -8.8$$

$$\hat{X} = a_{xy} + b_{xy}Y = -8.8 + .4Y$$

birth weight will be expected to increase by .4 pound. The
X-intercept obtained here is negative (-8.8). Although a negative value is not realistic for a variable such as birth weight,
it must be used here nevertheless in accordance with the computational procedures of regression analysis. Of course, although it is mathematically possible that a negative value will
sometimes be predicted for birth weight, such values should
be ignored for interpretive purposes. Furthermore it will be
inconvenient in this example to use the intercept as one of
the three plotted values to determine the location of the regression line on the scatter diagram.

Selecting three observed values for gestational age, 28, 32,
and 36, the predicted values for birth weight are computed as
follows:

$$\hat{X} = -8.8 + .4Y$$

$$\hat{X} = -8.8 + (.4)(28) = -8.8 + 11.2 = 2.4$$

$$\hat{X} = -8.8 + (.4)(32) = -8.8 + 12.8 = 4$$

$$\hat{X} = -8.8 + (.4)(36) = -8.8 + 14.4 = 5.6$$

Plotting the points where $Y = 28$, $X = 2.4$; $Y = 32$, $X = 4$;
and $Y = 36$, $X = 5.6$, the least-squares regression line is drawn
as displayed in Figure 13.7. Although this line looks very

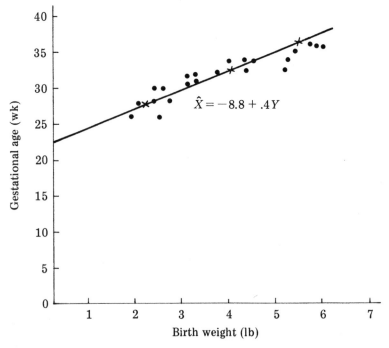

Figure 13.7.   Scatter diagram of birth weight and gestational age with
least-squares regression line for regression of birth weight on gestational
age.

Regression and Correlation

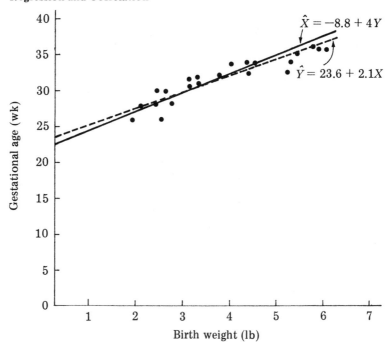

Figure 13.8. Comparison of least-squares regression lines for regression of gestational age on birth weight ($\hat{Y}$) and birth weight on gestational age ($\hat{X}$).

similar to the regression line in Figure 13.6, definite differences are observed upon close comparison, as displayed in Figure 13.8. Although both regression lines are fitted to the same set of observations, a different variable is being predicted in each case. Thus, in general, a different regression formula and line will apply for the regression of variable X on variable Y than for the regression of variable Y on variable X, because regression is an asymmetrical method of analysis.

Correlation Coefficient

Pearson's product moment correlation coefficient, which is symbolically represented by r, is a measure of association between two interval level sets of observations. The data requirements for a correlation analysis are the same as those for a least-squares regression analysis (i.e., interval level measurement, paired sets of observations, linearity, and homoscedasticity). Thus it is not appropriate to perform a correlation analysis with data for which a regression analysis is not appropriate.

Pearson's r indicates the direction and strength of an observed relationship, and ranges in value from -1.00 in the case of a perfect negative relationship to $+1.00$ for a perfect positive relationship, with *no* relationship being indicated by a value of zero. But, unlike the measures of association discussed in Chapter 12, Pearson's r cannot be given a PRE interpretation. The squared value of the correlation coefficient, r^2, is interpretable as a PRE measure, however. But, because a squared value is always positive, r^2 ranges in value from 0 to $+1.00$ and thus indicates the strength but not the direction of a relationship. Therefore both values, r and r^2, should be computed for a correlation analysis.

We will first present a conceptual discussion of the computation and interpretation of r^2. We will follow this by an example of the application of correlation analysis to the relationship between birth weight and gestational age. Finally we will present methods for testing the statistical significance of Pearson's r along with a discussion of the interpretation of a correlation analysis.

r^2 as a Proportional Reduction in Error Measure

In order to predict a value for every case in a distribution of observations on an interval level variable (Y), when given the distribution of observations on that variable only, the most successful method (prediction rule 1) would be to predict the mean of the distribution ($\overline{Y}$) for *each* observation. Prediction errors committed in such a situation may be measured as the sum of squared deviations about the mean of Y, which, as we know from Chapter 6, will always be minimum when computed about the mean. Therefore, $E_1 = \Sigma(Y - \overline{Y})^2$. Also, because the sum of squares is a measure of variation for an interval level variable, E_1 may be regarded as indicating the *total variation* in variable Y that a researcher would like to explain.

However, if information is available about another interval level variable (X), which is believed to be related to variable Y, prediction errors may be reduced by basing predictions of values for variable Y on the bivariate distribution of observations on both variables, X and Y. In this chapter we have learned a method for predicting values in exactly this kind of situation. The least-squares regression formula (prediction rule 2) is a method for predicting values for variable Y ($\hat{Y}$) based on the bivariate distribution of observations on both variables X and Y, so as to minimize prediction errors, which are measured as the sum of squared deviations about the least-squares regression line. Therefore $E_2 = \Sigma(Y - \hat{Y})^2$, which is a measure of the variation in variable Y that remains to be explained after information about variable X has been taken into consideration. Therefore E_2 may be regarded as indicating the *unexplained variation* in variable Y at this point.

By substituting these values for E_1 and E_2 in the general proportional reduction in error formula (PRE $= \dfrac{E_1 - E_2}{E_1}$), r^2 may be computed as

$$r^2 = \frac{\Sigma(Y - \overline{Y})^2 - \Sigma(Y - \hat{Y})^2}{\Sigma(Y - \overline{Y})^2} \qquad (13.7)$$

Therefore r^2 may be interpreted as indicating the proportional reduction in prediction error when predictions are based on the least-squares regression formula (or regression line) rather than on information about the distribution of variable Y ($\overline{Y}$) alone.

A more convenient and meaningful interpretation of r^2 is made possible, however, by conceptually reexpressing formula 13.7 as

$$r^2 = \frac{\text{Total Variation} - \text{Unexplained Variation}}{\text{Total Variation}} \qquad (13.8)$$

Furthermore, recognizing that total variation may be decomposed into explained and unexplained variation, that is,

Total Variation = Explained Variation + Unexplained Variation

and substituting in formula 13.8 we obtain

$$r^2 = \frac{(\text{Explained Variation} + \text{Unexplained Variation}) - \text{Unexplained Variation}}{\text{Total Variation}}$$

which reduces to

$$r^2 = \frac{\text{Explained Variation}}{\text{Total Variation}} \qquad (13.9)$$

Finally, by multiplying formula 13.9 by 100, r^2 is converted into a percentage and is interpretable as indicating the percentage of variation in one variable that is explained by another. Thus, when variable X is being used to predict values for variable Y, for example, r^2 indicates the percentage of variation in variable Y that is explained, or accounted for, by variable X. The stronger the relationship, the more useful will information about variable X be in predicting values for variable Y or explaining variation in Y, and the larger will be the value of r^2.

Computational Process

In computing Pearson's r^2 and r it is not possible to compute r^2 first and then determine r by finding $\sqrt{r^2}$, because we will not know whether to assign the value of r a positive or a negative sign (recall that r^2 will always be a positive value). Therefore we will proceed by first computing a value for r in such a way as to indicate whether the relationship is positive or negative and then determine the value for r^2 by squaring the value of r.

The correlation coefficient is computed according to the following formula:

$$r = \frac{N(\Sigma XY) - (\Sigma X)(\Sigma Y)}{\sqrt{[N(\Sigma X^2) - (\Sigma X)^2][N(\Sigma Y^2) - (\Sigma Y)^2]}} \qquad (13.10)$$

Although formula 13.10 appears quite formidable, most of the values for the computation of r should be available from previous computations. For example, if a least-squares regression analysis has already been performed, then the numerator of formula 13.10 is available; it is identical with the numerator of formula 13.2 for computing the slope of the regression line (b_{yx}). The denominator of formula 13.2 appears as the expression within the first set of brackets in the denominator of formula 13.10. Finally, the expressions within the second set of brackets in the denominator of formula 13.10, N, (ΣY^2), and ΣY (which is then squared), will be available from the computation of the mean and standard deviation of Y. Therefore in most cases the computation of r involves substituting a few readily available numbers in formula 13.10 and performing the necessary arithmetic. The value of r^2 is then obtained by squaring the value of r.

A Simple Example

In order to demonstrate the computation of r and r^2 let us return to the data regarding the ages of six pairs of siblings presented in Figure 13.4. Because all the observations lie exactly on the least-squares regression line as displayed in Figure 13.5, this relationship is a perfect positive one and therefore the values of both r and r^2 should equal $+1.00$. This may be verified by applying formula 13.10 as done in Table 13.6.

Note that the computations in Table 13.6 can be reduced considerably if we substitute the appropriate values from the computation for the least-squares regression line in Table 13.2. That is, from Table 13.2 we know that the numerator of formula 13.10 is $N(\Sigma XY) - (\Sigma X) - (\Sigma Y) = 210$, and for the denominator we know that $N(\Sigma X^2) - (\Sigma X)^2 = 105$, $N = 6$, and $\Sigma Y = 60$. Thus by substitution in formula 13.10 we have

$$r = \frac{210}{\sqrt{105[6(\Sigma Y^2) - 60^2]}}$$

which leaves us to find only (ΣY^2) before proceeding to solve for r. The reader should verify that when the value 670 is substituted for (ΣY^2) in this equation, a value of $+1.00$ is obtained for r.

Table 13.6. Computation of r and r^2 for Ages of Six Pairs of Siblings

X	Y	XY	X^2	Y^2
1	5	5	1	25
2	7	14	4	49
3	9	27	9	81
4	11	44	16	121
5	13	65	25	169
6	15	90	36	225
$\Sigma X = 21$	$\Sigma Y = 60$	$\Sigma XY = 245$	$\Sigma X^2 = 91$	$\Sigma Y^2 = 670$

$$r = \frac{N(\Sigma XY) - (\Sigma X)(\Sigma Y)}{\sqrt{[N(\Sigma X^2) - (\Sigma X)^2][N(\Sigma Y^2) - (\Sigma Y)^2]}}$$

$$r = \frac{6(245) - (21)(60)}{\sqrt{[6(91) - 21^2][6(670) - 60^2]}}$$

$$r = \frac{210}{\sqrt{(105)(420)}} = \frac{210}{\sqrt{44,100}} = \frac{210}{210} = +1.00$$

$$r^2 = 1.00^2 = 1.00$$

Birth Weight and Gestational Age

Table 13.7 gives the computation of r and r^2 for the data on birth weight and gestational age of 22 infants that were presented in Table 13.1. As in the previous example, these computations could also have been obtained by substitution of values from the least-squares regression analysis presented in Tables 13.3 and 13.5. Thus from Table 13.3 we know that the numerator of formula 13.10 is $N(\Sigma XY) - (\Sigma X)(\Sigma Y) = 1,803.5$ and in the denominator we have the expression $N(\Sigma X^2) - (\Sigma X)^2 = 846.1$. From Table 13.5 we know that the remaining expression in the denominator is $N(\Sigma Y^2) - (\Sigma Y)^2 = 4,485$. Thus we may solve for r as follows:

$$r = \frac{1803.5}{\sqrt{(846.1)(4485)}} = .93$$

Because Pearson's r (and r^2) is a symmetrical measure of association, it is not necessary to compute a separate value of r if we want to measure the strength of the relationship when birth weight is predicted from gestational age (as in the least-squares regression analysis presented in Table 13.5 and Figure 13.7). That is, regardless of whether birth weight is used to predict gestational age or gestational age is used to predict birth weight, the value of r is computed according

Table 13.7. Computation of r and r^2 for Birth Weight and Gestational Age

Birth weight (lb) X	Gestational age (wk) Y	XY	X^2	Y^2
1.9	26	49.4	3.6	676
2.1	28	58.8	4.4	784
2.5	28	70.0	6.2	784
2.5	30	75.0	6.2	900
2.6	30	78.0	6.8	900
2.6	26	67.6	6.8	676
2.8	28	78.4	7.8	784
3.1	32	99.2	9.6	1024
3.1	31	96.1	9.6	961
3.3	32	105.6	10.9	1024
3.3	31	102.3	10.9	961
3.8	32	121.6	14.4	1024
4.2	34	142.8	17.6	1156
4.6	34	156.4	21.2	1156
4.6	33	151.8	21.2	1089
4.8	34	163.2	23.0	1156
5.2	33	171.6	27.0	1089
5.3	34	180.2	28.1	1156
5.5	35	192.5	30.2	1225
5.8	36	208.8	33.6	1296
5.9	36	212.4	34.8	1296
6.2	36	223.2	38.4	1296
85.7	699	2804.9	372.3	22,413

$$r = \frac{N(\Sigma XY) - (\Sigma X)(\Sigma Y)}{\sqrt{[N(\Sigma X^2) - (\Sigma X)^2][N(\Sigma Y^2) - (\Sigma Y)^2]}}$$

$$r = \frac{22(2804.9) - (85.7)(699)}{\sqrt{[22(372.3) - 85.7^2][22(22,413) - 699^2]}}$$

$$r = \frac{1803.5}{\sqrt{(846.1)(4485)}} = \frac{1803.5}{1948} = .93$$

$r^2 = .93^2 = .86$

to formula 13.10 and is equal to .93 (and $r^2 = .86$) in both cases.

Testing the Significance of r

To test whether an observed value of r is statistically significant, that is, whether it is likely to be obtained by chance as a result of the random sampling process, the null hypothesis states that there is no relationship between variables X and Y ($H_0 : r = 0$). Either a one- or a two-tailed test may be applied.

When the number of observations is small, that is, when $N \leqslant 50$, the significance of r may be tested by a transformation to the t distribution according to the following formula:

$$t = \frac{r\sqrt{N-2}}{\sqrt{1-r^2}} \tag{13.11}$$

with df $= N - 2$

Thus for the relationship between birth weight and gestational age

$$t = \frac{.93\sqrt{20}}{\sqrt{1-.86}} = \frac{4.16}{.37} = 11.24$$

with df $= 20$

Referring to Table C.6 in Appendix C we see that a t value of 11.24 with 20 degrees of freedom for a one-tailed test is significant beyond the .001 level. Therefore the inference decision is to reject the null hypothesis; the value of r is statistically significant.

When the number of observations is large, that is, when $N > 50$, the significance of r may be tested by a transformation to the normal (z) distribution according to formula 13.12:

$$z = r\sqrt{N-1} \tag{13.12}$$

Table C.7 conveniently lists the minimum value of r that must be obtained for the .05 and .01 levels for one- and two-tailed tests for selected sample sizes. To use this table, locate the appropriate number of degrees of freedom (df $= N - 2$) in the first column, and then read across the corresponding row to find the minimum value of r required to reject the null hypothesis depending upon the level of significance and whether a one- or two-tailed test is used. For example, for birth weight and gestational age, $r = .93$ and df $= 20$. According to Table C.7 the minimum value of r that must be obtained to reject the null hypothesis at the .05 level for a one-tailed test with 20 degrees of freedom is .360. Because .93 exceeds this value, the inference decision is to reject the null hypothesis. Note that the null hypothesis would also be rejected at the .01 level in this case, because the minimum value of r at that level is .492.

It is not necessary to test the significance of r^2 directly.

If the observed value of r is found to be statistically significant, then it may be assumed that the corresponding value of r^2 is also significant.

Interpreting Correlations

Unlike the measures of association discussed in Chapter 12, a correlation analysis does not yield a single value that adequately indicates both the direction and the strength of a relationship. Instead, two values must be considered: r and r^2.

The most often reported result from a correlation analysis is the correlation coefficient, r, which may range in value from -1.00 in the case of a perfect negative relationship to $+1.00$ in the case of a perfect positive relationship and will equal zero when no relationship is displayed. By itself, however, r is primarily useful for indicating the direction and testing the statistical significance of a relationship. Although many researchers also consider the size of r to indicate the strength of a relationship, this can be seriously misleading unless great caution is exercised.

At first it is tempting to interpret the strength of a correlation coefficient according to the guidelines presented in Figure 12.1, and indeed many researchers do just that. But it is not appropriate to evaluate r in this manner, because Figure 12.1 is designed to interpret only PRE measures, and r is not one. However, r^2, which is conveniently and directly derived from r, is a PRE measure and thus provides a means for interpreting the results of a correlation analysis according to Figure 12.1. But because the value of r^2 may range from 0 to $+1.00$ and will never be negative, r^2 does not indicate the direction of a relationship. Therefore both r and r^2 must be considered when interpreting the results of a correlation analysis in terms of both direction and strength.

To appreciate why it may be misleading to evaluate the strength of a relationship according to the value for r, consider Table 13.8. A good rule of thumb in evaluating the strength of any relationship is that a "strong" relationship is one in which at least a simple majority, or 50 percent, of the variation in one variable is explained by the other. Applying this rule and referring to Table 13.8, we see that rather high values of r may occur when much less than 50 percent of the variation is explained. For example, when $r = .50$, 25 percent of the variation is explained; when $r = .60$, 36 percent of the variation is explained; and even when r is as high as .70 only 49 percent of the variation is explained. Thus r must be greater than .70 before at least 50 percent of the variation is explained. As can also been seen in Table 13.8, r^2 is a more reliable indicator of the strength of a relationship, because the value of r^2 directly corresponds to the percentage of variation explained, which is computed by

Table 13.8. r^2 and Percentage of Variation Explained for Selected Values of r

r	r^2	Variation explained (%)
.10	.01	1
.15	.02	2
.20	.04	4
.25	.06	6
.30	.09	9
.35	.12	12
.40	.16	16
.45	.20	20
.50	.25	25
.55	.30	30
.60	.36	36
.65	.42	42
.70	.49	49
.75	.56	56
.80	.64	64
.85	.72	72
.90	.81	81
.95	.90	90
1.00	1.00	100

multiplying r^2 by 100. On the other hand the relationship between r and the percentage of variation explained is not linear, as demonstrated in Figure 13.9. When working with sample data, however, a test for statistical significance must be performed regardless of the percentage of variation explained, because even when this percentage is as large as 80 percent or 90 percent, for example, r may not be statistically significant.

Another point to keep in mind in interpreting the results of a correlation analysis is that r and r^2 are symmetrical measures. That is, the values for r and r^2 that are computed when variable X is used to predict values for variable Y will also apply when variable Y is used to predict values for variable X. For this reason a correlation analysis may *not* be interpreted as demonstrating a causal relationship. That is, the observation of a very strong correlation between two variables is not sufficient evidence to establish that variable X is the cause of variable Y, because exactly the same values of r and r^2 will be obtained to support the opposite interpretation that variable Y is the cause of variable X. For example, it might be expected that there is a high positive correlation between the amount of time a nurse spends with a patient and patient recovery rate. If this high correlation is found, it

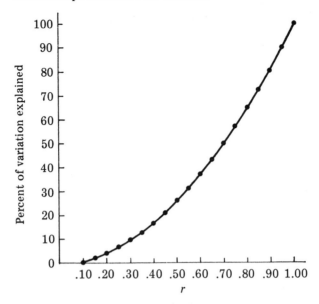

Figure 13.9. Values of *r* and percent of variation explained.

might be interpreted as demonstrating that an increase in the amount of time a nurse spends with a patient causes an increase in the patient's recovery rate. But although this interpretation appears logically sound, it should be remembered that an identical high positive correlation will also be found between patient recovery rate and the amount of time a nurse spends with the patient. This result might be interpreted as demonstrating that an increase in patient recovery rate causes an increase in the amount of time a nurse spends with a patient, because patients who are in a better state of health are better able to interact with others, and this encourages a nurse to spend an increased amount of time with such patients. On the other hand, patients who are slow to recover encourage less interaction, the extreme case being terminally ill patients whom nurses may tend to avoid, either consciously or unconsciously, because such cases are difficult and upsetting. Thus, equally plausible but opposite interpretations are sometimes possible for a single correlation analysis.

Correlations Between More Than Two Variables

Researchers are often interested in studying more than two interval level variables and therefore may perform a correlation analysis for each combination of variables, taking them two at a time. For example, a researcher interested in blood pressure, pulse, respiration, and temperature may perform six correlation analyses by combining them as follows:

1. Blood pressure and pulse
2. Blood pressure and respiration

3. Blood pressure and temperature
4. Pulse and respiration
5. Pulse and temperature
6. Respiration and temperature

Such results are typically reported in summary fashion by presenting a table, called a *correlation matrix*, which provides a cross-listing of the correlation coefficients computed between all pairs of variables. Table 13.9 is an example of one method of presenting a correlation matrix. Reading across the rows, the first row contains the correlation coefficient (r) computed between blood pressure and each variable. Similarly the second row contains the correlation coefficients for pulse, the third row for respiration, and the fourth row for temperature. The significance level for each correlation is indicated by the use of asterisks as appropriate. The absence of an asterisk indicates that a correlation is not significant. Thus we can see that blood pressure has a very strong positive correlation with pulse ($r = .92; p < .01$), a moderately strong positive correlation with respiration ($r = .65; p < .05$), and no significant correlation with temperature ($r = .46$). Similarly pulse has a significant and strong positive correlation with each of the other measures: blood pressure ($r = .92; p < .01$), respiration ($r = .78; p < .05$), and temperature ($r = .84; p < .01$).

A closer examination of Table 13.9 reveals several important features of a correlation matrix that are highlighted in Table 13.10. First, notice that each of the values in the cells that lie diagonally from the upper left corner to the lower right corner, called the *major diagonal* of a correlation matrix, is equal to $+1.00$. This is because these cells contain the correlation of each variable with itself, and this would logically be a perfect positive correlation with $r = +1.00$. Also there are two groups of cells located off the major diagonal, one above and one below, as outlined by the triangles in Table 13.10. It is important to recognize that these cells contain identical information. For example, both groups contain the correlation

Table 13.9. Pearson Correlation Matrix for Four Physiological Variables

Variable	Blood pressure	Pulse	Respiration	Temperature
Blood pressure (B.P.)	1.00**	.92**	.65*	.46
Pulse	.92**	1.00**	.78*	.84**
Respiration	.65*	.78*	1.00**	.70*
Temperature	.46	.84**	.70*	1.00**

* $p < .05$
** $p < .01$

Table 13.10. Partitioned Pearson Correlation Matrix for Four
Physiological Variables

Variable	Blood pressure	Pulse	Respiration	Temperature
Blood pressure	1.00**	.92**	.65*	.46
Pulse	.92**	1.00**	.78*	.84**
Respiration	.65*	.78*	1.00**	.70*
Temperature	.46	.84**	.70*	1.00**

* $p < .05$
** $p < .01$

between blood pressure and pulse ($r = .92$), the correlation
between pulse and temperature ($r = .84$), and so on. Furthermore, although it was initially determined that a total of only
six correlation coefficients could be computed for four measures combined two at a time, Table 13.9 is a 4 × 4 table and
includes 16 cells containing coefficients. This is because Table
13.9 includes much unnecessary and/or redundant information. Specifically it is of no use to display the correlations
that lie on the major diagonal, because researchers are not interested in the correlation for a variable with itself, which will
always equal +1.00. Also, because identical information is
contained in the cells located above and below the major diagonal, Table 13.9 includes needless repetition. Therefore the
correlation matrix presented in Table 13.9 may be greatly
simplified by eliminating the correlations on the major diagonal and one set of correlations off the major diagonal, as
shown in Table 13.11, which includes only the six correlation
coefficients located above the major diagonal. This is the
standard format for presenting a correlation matrix in the research literature, because it includes all the important information while excluding useless and/or redundant correlations,
making the matrix much quicker and easier to read. A similar
matrix may be used to present other measures of association,

Table 13.11. Simplified Pearson Correlation Matrix for Four
Physiological Variables

Variable	Pulse	Respiration	Temperature
Blood pressure	.92**	.65*	.46
Pulse		.78*	.84**
Respiration			.70*

* $p < .05$
** $p < .01$

such as lambda, gamma, Somers' d, and Kendall's tau, as well.

Another approach to analyzing more than two variables is *multiple regression and correlation*. Basically this multivariate procedure, which is beyond the scope of an introductory text, allows a researcher to examine how well two or more independent variables, when their influence is considered simultaneously, may be used to predict values for a single dependent variable. For example, as part of an effort to assess the validity of a patient anxiety scale, a researcher may be interested in how well all four physiological measures included in Table 13.9, considered in combination, predict values on the scale.

Other Correlation Methods

There are several correlational procedures in addition to Pearson's correlation coefficient. These other procedures are applied when the data do not conform to all the basic requirements for a Pearson correlation analysis. For example, a commonly used method for performing a correlation analysis for a nonlinear relationship is the computation of the *correlation ratio*, called eta squared (η^2). When either or both variables are measured at the ordinal level, one of two methods is commonly used. *Kendall's rank order correlation coefficient* (tau) was discussed in Chapter 12. An alternative procedure is *Spearman's rank order correlation coefficient*, called rho (ρ). While Kendall's tau measures the relative preponderance of same- vs. reverse-ordered pairs, Spearman's rho measures the extent to which there is agreement between two sets of rank-ordered observations.

WORKING WITH AND INTERPRETING DATA

Table 1. Age and Percentage of RDA Caloric Intake

Age	%RDA
23	102
56	79
60	78
37	85
24	88
20	90
30	90
43	85
64	70
60	70
65	64
40	80
45	76
72	60
70	65

1. Plot a scatter diagram for the data presented in Table 1, and evaluate the linearity, scedasticity, direction, and strength of the relationship.

2. Compute the least-squares regression formula, and fit the regression line to your scatter diagram.

3. Compute Pearson's correlation coefficient, r, and r^2.

4. Test the correlation for statistical significance using formula 13.11, then verify your result according to Table C.7.

5. Interpret the results of the regression and correlation analysis you performed in questions 1 through 4 in terms of the direction, strength, and significance of the relationship between age and percentage of RDA caloric intake.

6. What would you predict as the percentage of RDA caloric intake for a person who is 27 years old?

7. If a person is 30 years old and has a 90% RDA caloric intake, by how much would you expect that person's percent RDA caloric intake to increase or decrease by age 40? Specify the *amount* and *direction* of the expected change.

8. The authors of the following articles report Pearson correlation coefficients among their findings. For each article, evaluate the appropriateness of the author's use of this technique. Describe and interpret these findings, and compare your conclusions with those of the author.

   Christensen, Mark G., Carla A.B. Lee, and Phillip W. Bugg. Professional development of nurse practitioners as a function of need motivation, learning style, and locus of control. *Nursing Research* 28:51–56, 1979. See Table 6.
   Davitz, Lois Jean, and Sidney Harrison Pendleton. Nurses' inferences of suffering. *Nursing Research* 18:100–107, 1969. See Table 7.
   Johnson, Jean E., James M. Dabbs, Jr., and Howard Leventhal. Psychological factors in the welfare of surgical patients. *Nursing Research* 19:18–29, 1970. See Table 7.

Statistics in Perspective

Statistics as a Tool

We have attempted to present statistics as a convenient and useful tool that is available to the researcher for the purpose of examining data and communicating findings but that must be applied in combination with logic and careful thought. Although much of the utility and power of a statistical analysis is derived directly from the mathematical principles upon which it is based, numbers are meaningless by themselves. They are of use to a researcher only when they are identified as measurements of a variable of interest and importance. Therefore it is essential not to become involved in the mathematical and computational aspects of a statistical analysis to the extent of losing sight of the original purpose of the investigation. That is, the analysis is performed to answer a specific research question, not to generate a collection of numbers devoid of interpretation.

Statistics may aid a researcher in arriving at logical conclusions in answer to a research question but should never be allowed to substitute for original and creative thought regarding the interpretation, implications, and application of research findings. This is not to say, however, that the researcher has freedom to suggest interpretations and applications that are not supported by the data. Although it is often said that statistics can be used to support any idea or interpretation, this is not true. It is true, however, that statistics may be presented, intentionally or unintentionally, in such a way as to mislead not only others but even the researcher him- or herself. This is well demonstrated in Huff's witty little book, *How To Lie With Statistics.* In most cases "lying with statistics" is a result of inappropriate application of a statistical technique to an analysis problem, but it may also result from erroneous computations or incomplete reporting of the results of the analysis. Misuses of statistics occur even in articles published in professional journals, although most journals try to detect such misuse in their manuscript review process. Thus the fact that something appears in print should not be taken as a guarantee that it is correct. Both researcher and consumer must clearly understand the data requirements, applications, and limitations of statistical techniques to avoid being misled by wrong application of this tool.

Selection of an Appropriate Statistical Technique

The purpose of a research investigation is an important determinant of the statistical analysis to be applied. As reflected by the organization of this text, different techniques are available depending upon whether the focus of the investigation is on description, on the examination of differences, or on the examination of relationships. But no matter what the purpose of a research investigation, there still remain a great many statistical techniques that might be chosen for the analysis. The decision as to which of these is most appropriate for a given situation will most often depend upon the nature of the data the researcher has collected.

As we have seen, each statistical technique makes specific assumptions or requirements about the nature of the data to be analyzed. In general the most important of these is the level of measurement (i.e., nominal, ordinal, or interval). Some techniques may be applied to all levels of measurement, while others require that the data be measured on either the ordinal or the interval level, and still others require that the data be measured at the interval level. A good general rule is to select the technique that will make the maximum use of the information available in the data. The first choice usually is to apply an interval level technique if possible, the next choice is for an ordinal level technique, and nominal level techniques are employed when no other choice is available.

Many people claim to have a natural aversion to statistics and data analysis. Such an attitude is probably due to ignorance more than to anything else. But regardless of how much time, thought, effort, and skill the researcher invests in defining a research problem, designing and selecting a sample, developing a measurement tool, and collecting the data, all of these are wasted and the research question left unanswered unless the data are adequately analyzed and interpreted. Furthermore the analysis should be planned early in the research design stage of a study, so that provision may be made for the collection of data appropriate to the desired and perhaps necessary statistical techniques. It is usually too late to consider analysis strategies after data collection is completed; and it is rarely fruitful for a researcher to go on a "fishing trip" with data in hand to see what kinds of interesting or useful results may be teased out of the data by using every statistical technique imaginable until something significant is uncovered.

Statistical vs. Substantive Significance

Even when an analysis using a technique appropriate to the data and problem under study is carefully and accurately conducted and reported, it is almost never to be regarded as conclusive. As was emphasized in the discussion of the logic of inferential statistics and hypothesis testing, statistics do not enable a researcher to *prove* anything. At best they may be considered to lend support to a particular interpretation. The inevitable limitations and shortcomings of *any* research investigation require that findings, no matter how impressive, be verified by replication with different subjects, in different settings, at different times, and by different investigators. Such replication is especially important before critical decisions are made on the basis of research findings—such as modifications in patient care plans, distribution of personnel, and allocation of resources.

Therefore it is important to distinguish between the *statistical* and the *substantive* significance of research findings. If an analysis of a well-designed and well-conducted study reveals results that are statistically significant, it is then necessary to ask, "So what?" This is because, given precise measurement instruments and a large number of observations, differences or relationships that are relatively small in magnitude may nevertheless pass the test for statistical significance. Such findings may not be sufficiently large or strong to elicit important action in response, however. There are no standard tests or formats for evaluating the substantive significance of research findings. Each individual must make his or her own assessment of the value of a research finding in terms of how that information may be used. Such an evaluation usually is arrived at by weighing the potential benefits to be derived from taking certain actions against the potential costs or risks associated with those actions. Generally an action is taken when the benefits are judged to sufficiently outweigh the costs and risks. Thus there may be instances in which substantive significance is of much greater importance than statistical significance. Decisions involving patient care, in which the risks are extreme in terms of life and death, are an obvious example.

Final Note

Many people wrongly think of statistics as a static collection of formulas and numbers. But as a field of study, statistics has advanced tremendously during the last 50 years—especially since World War II, when the federal government became actively involved in promoting and supporting research in many disciplines. The growth and development of statistics are expected to continue, with no apparent end in sight.

It is therefore obviously impossible to provide comprehensive coverage of the entire field of statistics in a single book. The number of statistical techniques that could not be included in this book vastly outnumber those that are. Furthermore it is not possible, especially in an introductory text, to cover everything there is to know about each statistical method that is included. Therefore on completion of this book you should not be deceived into thinking that you know everything there is to know about statistics. Instead you have received an introductory exposure to several of the most common basic statistical concepts and techniques. Indeed, your knowledge of statistics has only just begun.

Reference

Huff, Darrell. *How To Lie With Statistics.* New York: Norton, 1954.

Bibliography

Introductory Texts

Anderson, Theodore R., and Morris Zelditch, Jr. *A Basic Course in Statistics with Sociological Applications.* New York: Holt, Rinehart & Winston, 1975.

Blalock, Hubert M., Jr. *Social Statistics.* New York: McGraw-Hill, 1960.

Blalock, Hubert M., Jr. *Social Statistics.* 2d ed. New York: McGraw-Hill, 1972.

Colton, Theodore. *Statistics in Medicine.* Boston: Little, Brown and Company, 1974.

Dixon, Wilfred J., and Frank J. Massey. *Introduction to Statistical Analysis.* New York: McGraw-Hill, 1957.

Downey, Kenneth J. *Elementary Social Statistics.* New York: Random House, 1975.

Dunn, Olive Jean. *Basic Statistics: A Primer for the Biomedical Sciences.* New York: John Wiley & Sons, 1964.

Freund, John E. *Modern Elementary Statistics.* Englewood Cliffs, New Jersey: Prentice-Hall, 1973.

Gehring, Robert E. *Basic Behavioral Statistics.* Boston: Houghton Mifflin, 1978.

Kilpatrick, S. James, Jr. *Statistical Principles in Health Care Information.* Baltimore: University Park Press, 1973.

Korin, Basil P. *Statistical Concepts for the Social Sciences.* Cambridge, Mass.: Winthrop, 1975.

Levin, Jack. *Elementary Statistics in Social Research.* New York: Harper & Row, 1977.

Loether, Herman J., and Donald G. McTavish. *Descriptive Statistics for Sociologists: An Introduction.* Boston: Allyn and Bacon, 1974a.

Loether, Herman J., and Donald G. McTavish. *Inferential Statistics for Sociologists: An Introduction.* Boston: Allyn and Bacon, 1974b.

Leonard, Wilbert Marcellus, II. *Basic Social Statistics.* St. Paul: West, 1976.

Mueller, John H., Karl F. Schuessler, and Herbert L. Costner. *Statistical Reasoning in Sociology.* Boston: Houghton Mifflin, 1970.

Mueller, John H., Karl F. Schuessler, and Herbert L. Costner. *Statistical Reasoning in Sociology.* Boston: Houghton Mifflin, 1977.

Ott, Lyman, William Mendenhall, and Richard F. Larson. *Statistics: A Tool for the Social Sciences.* North Scituate, Massachusetts: Duxbury Press, 1978.

Sokal, Robert R., and F. James Rohlf. *Introduction to Biostatistics.* San Francisco: W. H. Freeman, 1973.

Walker, Helen M. *Mathematics Essential for Elementary Statistics.* New York: Holt, Rinehart & Winston, 1951.

Weiss, Robert S. *Statistics in Social Research: An Introduction.* New York: John Wiley & Sons, 1968.

Zeisel, Hans. *Say It With Figures.* New York: Harper & Row, 1968.

Advanced and Special Topics

Amick, Daniel J., and Herbert Walberg (eds.). *Introductory Multivariate Analysis.* Berkeley, Calif.: McCutchan, 1975.

Bradley, James. V. *Distribution-Free Statistical Tests.* Englewood Cliffs, New Jersey: Prentice-Hall, 1968.

Conover, W.J. *Practical Nonparametric Statistics.* New York: John Wiley & Sons, 1971.

Cooley, William W. and Paul R. Lohnes. *Multivariate Data Analysis.* New York: John Wiley & Sons, 1971.

Costner, Herbert L. Criteria for Measures of Association. *American Sociological Review,* Vol. 30 (June): 341–353, 1965.

Daniel, Wayne W. *Applied Nonparametric Statistics.* Boston: Houghton Mifflin, 1978.

Freeman, Linton C. *Elementary Applied Statistics: For Students in Behavioral Science.* New York: John Wiley & Sons, 1965.

Hays, William L. *Statistics.* New York: Holt, Rinehart & Winston, 1963.

Kerlinger, Fred N., and Elazar J. Pedhazur. *Multiple Regression in Behavioral Research.* New York: Holt, Rinehart & Winston, 1973.

Mosteller, Frederick, and Robert E. K. Rourke. *Sturdy Statistics: Nonparametrics and Order Statistics.* Reading, Mass.: Addison-Wesley, 1973.

Reynolds, H.T. *The Analysis of Cross-Classifications.* New York: The Free Press, 1977.

Schuessler, Karl. *Analyzing Social Data.* Boston: Houghton Mifflin, 1971.

Siegel, Sidney. *Nonparametric Statistics: For the Behavioral Sciences.* New York: McGraw-Hill, 1956.

Somers, Robert H. On the Measurement of Association. *American Sociological Review,* Vol. 33 (April): 291–292, 1968.

Tatsuoka, Maurice M. *Multivariate Analysis.* New York: John Wiley & Sons, 1971.

Winer, B.J. *Statistical Principles in Experimental Design.* New York: McGraw-Hill, 1971.

Appendixes

Review of Mathematical Operations

Although this book does not take a highly mathematical approach to the subject of statistics, competence in *elementary* arithmetic and algebraic operations is essential to understanding and performing the techniques discussed. The discussions in this appendix are brief and are intended as a review rather than as an introduction to new material. A reader who desires more intensive coverage of any of these operations should consult a basic algebra text (such as Walker, 1951). An understanding of the operations discussed here will be adequate for the purposes of this book, however. Modern calculators are able to perform most of these operations. But while these machines are extremely useful tools, the reader is cautioned against using them as a substitute for thinking and learning.

Conventions of Expressing Multiplication

The basic rules of addition, subtraction, multiplication, and division will not be reviewed, as they are assumed to be well known. It should be recalled, however, that multiplication may be indicated by the symbol $\times$ or $\cdot$ or by the separation of numbers by parentheses. Thus, "5 multiplied by 2" may be indicated in any of the following ways:

2×5

$2 \cdot 5$

$2(5)$

$(2)(5)$

Also, when a letter is used to symbolize a number, multiplication is indicated by simply placing a number or another letter adjacent to it. Thus, "a multiplied by 2" is indicated as $2a$, and "a multiplied by b" is indicated as ab.

Operations Involving Zero

A number is not changed by the addition or subtraction of zero. Thus, $5 + 0 = 5$, and $5 - 0 = 5$. However, addition to or subtraction from zero results in a new value. Thus, $0 + 2 = 2$, and $0 - 2 = -2$.

Whenever zero is involved in the process of multiplication, the resulting product is *always* zero. Thus, $36 \times 0 = 0$, and $0 \times 54 = 0$.

Whenever zero is divided by any number, the resulting

quotient is *always* zero. Thus, $0/12 = 0$ and $0/246 = 0$. However, *numbers cannot be divided by zero*, because the resulting quotient is infinite and is therefore said to be undefined in mathematics. Thus, it is *not possible* to perform operations such as $6/0$, $55/0$, or $0/0$.

Also, for purposes of rounding (see Chapter 2), zero is considered to be an *even* number.

Signed Numbers

A number may be assigned either a positive ($+$) or a negative ($-$) sign to indicate whether it is located to the right or to the left of zero along the number scale, with positive numbers located to the right and negative numbers to the left of zero:

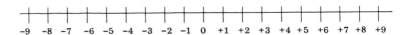

Regardless of magnitude, negative numbers are considered smaller in value than positive numbers and zero. Thus, -6 is smaller in value than 0, $+1$, or $+5$. Also, the larger the magnitude of a negative number, the smaller is its value. Thus, -8 is smaller than -7, -4, or -1.

The *absolute value* of a signed number is indicated by the placement of the number between two vertical bars, which indicate that the sign of the number is to be ignored (in other words, the number is to be treated as a positive number regardless of whether its sign is $+$ or $-$). Thus, $|4| = 4$ and $|-4| = 4$.

For calculations involving only positive numbers, the standard rules of addition, subtraction, multiplication, and division apply. However, a few basic rules must be remembered when one or more negative numbers are included in calculations, as described in the following section.

Operations Involving Negative Numbers
Addition

To add a group of negative numbers, determine the sum of their absolute values and place a *negative* sign in front of their sum. Thus, $(-5) + (-3) = -8$ and $(-12) + (-4) + (-5) = -21$.

To add a positive number and negative number, ignore their signs and subtract the smaller number from the larger number, then place the sign of the larger number in front of the difference you have obtained. Thus

$$(-40) + 32 = |-40| - |32| = -8$$

$$(-13) + 20 = |20| - |-13| = +7$$

$$16 + (-18) = |-18| - |16| = -2$$

$$20 + (-15) = |20| - |-15| = +5$$

To add a series of positive and negative numbers, group all positive numbers together and all negative numbers together and sum each group. Then add their sums by subtracting the smaller sum from the larger sum and placing the sign of the larger sum in front of the difference obtained. For example:

$$(-3) + (-2) + 5 + (-6) + 4 = [(-3) + (-2) + (-6)] + (5 + 4)$$
$$= (-11) + 9 = -2$$
$$(-4) + 7 + (-2) + 3 + 6 + (-1) = [(-4) + (-2) + (-1)]$$
$$+ (7 + 3 + 6) = (-7) + 16 = 9$$

Subtraction
To subtract one number from another when either or both numbers are negative, change the sign of the number being subtracted and then proceed as in addition. Thus,

$$6 - (-2) = 6 + 2 = 8$$

$$(-6) - (-2) = (-6) + 2 = -4$$

$$(-6) - 2 = (-6) + (-2) = -8$$

Multiplication
Two basic rules apply for the multiplication of signed numbers. First, when two numbers with the *same sign* are multiplied, the sign of the product is always *positive.* Thus,

$$3 \times 5 = 15$$

$$(-3) \times (-5) = 15$$

Second, when two numbers with *different signs* are multiplied the product is always *negative.* Thus,

$$3 \times (-5) = -15$$

$$(-3) \times 5 = -15$$

Also, when more than two numbers all with positive signs are multiplied, the sign of the product is always positive. Thus,

$$2 \times 4 \times 3 = 24$$

However, when more than two numbers are multiplied, one or more of which have a negative sign, the sign of the product will be positive if there is an *even* number of negative signs and negative if there is an *odd* number of negative signs. Thus,

$$2 \times (-4) \times (-3) = +24 \qquad (-2) \times 4 \times 3 = -24$$

$$(-2) \times (-4) \times 3 = +24 \qquad 2 \times (-4) \times 3 = -24$$

$$(-2) \times 4 \times (-3) = +24 \qquad 2 \times 4 \times (-3) = -24$$

$$(-2) \times (-4) \times (-3) = -24$$

Division

The same rules apply for the division of signed numbers as for multiplication. For example,

$$15/3 = 5$$

$$(-15)/(-3) = 5$$

$$15/(-3) = -5$$

$$(-15)/3 = -5$$

Operations Involving Fractions

Addition and Subtraction

Before fractions may be added or subtracted it is necessary to determine a *common denominator*. Although it is not always the most efficient method, conversion to a common denominator may be accomplished by multiplying both the numerator and the denominator of one fraction by the denominator of the other, and vice versa. Fractions may then be combined by adding or subtracting their numerators. Thus,

$$2/3 + 5/6 = 12/18 + 15/18 = 27/18 = 1\ 9/18 = 1\ 1/2$$

$$3/4 - 5/8 = 24/32 - 20/32 = 4/32 = 1/8$$

Note that it is customary to *reduce* fractions as in the foregoing examples, in which 27/18 was reduced to 1 1/2 and 4/32 was reduced to 1/8.

Multiplication

A separate product is determined for the numerators and a separate product is determined for the denominators, for example,

$$\frac{1}{2} \times \frac{3}{4} = \frac{3}{8} \text{ and } \frac{2}{3} \times \frac{5}{6} = \frac{10}{18} = \frac{5}{9}$$

Division

Invert the *divisor* (the fraction by which another is being divided) and proceed as in multiplication, for example,

$$\frac{2}{5} \div \frac{1}{3} = \frac{2}{5} \times \frac{3}{1} = \frac{6}{5} = 1\frac{1}{5}$$

It is also important to remember that the quotient of any number divided by itself is equal to 1. Thus, $3/3 = 1$ and $12/12 = 1$. Of course, this does not apply to zero, and $0/0$ is undefined.

Simplifying Fractions

Fractions may be simplified by one of two procedures. First, common terms in both numerator and denominator may be *canceled*, because their quotient is equal to 1. Thus we may simplify the following fraction which is expressed algebraically:

$$\frac{ac}{bc} = \frac{a\cancel{c}}{b\cancel{c}} = \frac{a}{b}$$

Second, fractions may be simplified by multiplying both numerator and denominator by a common factor. Thus,

$$\frac{a}{b/c} = \frac{ac}{(\cancel{c})b/\cancel{c}} = \frac{ac}{b} \text{ and } \frac{a/c}{b} = \frac{(\cancel{c})a/\cancel{c}}{bc} = \frac{a}{bc}$$

Conversion of Fractions to Decimals

Another method of simplifying a fraction is to convert it into a decimal number by dividing the numerator by the denominator. For example,

$$\frac{2}{5} = .4 \qquad \frac{1}{3} = .33 \qquad \frac{1}{2} = .5 \qquad \frac{3}{4} = .75 \qquad \frac{9}{10} = .9$$

In fact, this is how fractions are usually handled in statistics because decimals are generally much easier to work with in computation.

Operations Involving Decimals

Addition and Subtraction

The addition and subtraction of decimals follow the same rules as the addition and subtraction of whole numbers. The main thing to remember is that the decimal points must be aligned directly above and below one another. A good rule to follow is to write each number so that it occupies the same number of places to the right of the decimal point. This is done by adding nonsignificant zeros wherever necessary. Thus the addition 2.03 + 41.6 + 7.265 is performed as follows:

```
 2.030
41.600
 7.265
------
50.895
```

Similarly the subtraction 59.5 − 2.33 is performed as

```
 59.50
− 2.33
------
 57.17
```

Multiplication

The multiplication of decimals follows the basic rules for multiplication of whole numbers. The main thing to remember when working with decimals is that the product contains as many places to the right of the decimal point as there are in the numbers that were multiplied to obtain that product *combined*. For example, $12.63 \times 2.5 = 31.575$, and $1.5 \times 3.3 \times 2.7 = 13.365$.

Division

If the divisor is expressed in decimals it is necessary first to move the decimal point as many places to the right as possible in order to convert the divisor to a whole number. The decimal point in the dividend (even if it is a whole number) must then be moved the same number of places to the right as was done with the divisor. For example,

$$3.28\overline{)51.496} = 328\overline{)5149.6}^{\,15.7}$$

$$5.5\overline{)176} = 55\overline{)1760}^{\,32}$$

$$3.6\overline{)63} = 36\overline{)630.0} \quad \overset{17.5}{\phantom{36\overline{)630.0}}}$$

Proportions and Percentages

One way of thinking about fractions is that they express one number (the numerator) as a part of a larger number or whole (the denominator). When fractions are converted to decimals by means of division, the resulting decimal may also be considered as a *proportion.* That is, a proportion is a decimal number that indicates what part of a whole is represented by a smaller quantity, as computed by the following formula:

$$P = \frac{n}{N}$$

where P = a proportion

n = number of items or observations in a subgroup

N = total number of items or observations

For example, if a group of 50 patients is composed of 30 females and 20 males, the size of each patient subgroup by sex may be expressed as a proportion:

Females   *Males*

$$P = \frac{n}{N} = \frac{30}{50} = .60 \qquad P = \frac{n}{N} = \frac{20}{50} = .40$$

Note that the sum of the proportions for all subgroups is always equal to 1.00, thus, .60 + .40 = 1.00.

But in statistics it is often more useful to convert a proportion into a *percentage* by multiplying it by 100, as indicated in the following formula:

$$\% = \frac{n}{N}\,(100)$$

where   % = a percentage

n = number of items or observations in a subgroup

N = total number of items or observations

Thus, the data regarding the number of female and male patients may be converted into percentages, as follows:

Females

$$\% = \frac{n}{N}(100) = \frac{30}{50}(100) = .60\,(100) = 60\%$$

Males

$$\% = \frac{n}{N}(100) = \frac{20}{50}(100) = .40\,(100) = 40\%$$

Note that a quick method for converting any decimal into a percentage is simply to move the decimal point two places to the right. This is the equivalent of multiplying by 100. Also, the sum of the percentages for all subgroups is always equal to 100%, thus, 60% + 40% = 100%.

Operations with Algebraic Equations
Grouping
Algebraic expressions are often grouped by the use of parentheses (), brackets [], and braces { }, which indicate that the expressions within them are to be treated as a single value or quantity. The rule when working with such grouped expressions is to perform the operations within parentheses first, within the brackets second, and within the braces third, working from the innermost groupings outward. For example,

$$\{[5(2 + 3)] - [2(4 + 1)]\} + 3(5 - 2)$$
$$= \{[5(5)] - [2(5)]\} + 3(3)$$
$$= \{25 - 10\} + 9$$
$$= 15 + 9$$
$$= 24$$

Algebraic Order
Another important algebraic rule is that multiplication and division must be performed before addition and subtraction unless grouping signs indicate otherwise. For example,

$3(5) - 2 = 15 - 2 = 13$	*not*	$3(5) - 2 = 3(3) = 9$
$2 + 3(2) = 2 + 6 = 8$	*not*	$2 + 3(2) = 5(2) = 10$
$10 - 6/2 = 10 - 3 = 7$	*not*	$10 - 6/2 = 4/2 = 2$
$24/8 + 4 = 3 + 4 = 7$	*not*	$24/8 + 4 = 24/12 = 2$

Collecting Terms

A useful method for simplifying an algebraic equation is to collect, or group, common terms within the equation. For example,

$2x + 3y + 3x = z$ may be simplified as $(2x + 3x) + 3y = z$

$$5x + 3y = z$$

$5x + 2y - 6y - 2x = z$ may be simplified as

$$(5x - 2x) + (2y - 6y) = z$$

$$3x - 4y = z$$

Substitution

It is sometimes useful to substitute a single term by a larger, more complex expression that will then allow for simplification. For example,

Given $\dfrac{a - b}{2} = c$

if $a = d + b$

then $\dfrac{(d + b) - b}{2} = c$

and $\dfrac{d}{2} = c$

Manipulating Equations

The main rule to remember when manipulating equations is that, in order to maintain the equality, whatever operation is performed on one side of the equals sign must also be performed on the other side. The most common purpose for manipulating an equation is to "solve" it by isolating a single quantity or term of interest. The following examples demonstrate the use of addition, subtraction, multiplication, and division in solving a simple equation for X.

Addition: $X - 2 = 5$

$$X - 2 + 2 = 5 + 2$$

$$X = 7$$

Subtraction: $X + 3 = 8$

$$X + 3 - 3 = 8 - 3$$

$$X = 5$$

Multiplication: $\dfrac{X}{2} = 6$

$$2\left(\dfrac{X}{2}\right) = 2\,(6)$$

$$X = 12$$

Division: $4X = 24$

$$\dfrac{4X}{4} = \dfrac{24}{4}$$

$$X = 6$$

Squares and Square Roots

When a number is multiplied by itself, a superscript number (called an *exponent*) is affixed to it which designates how many times the number is to be multiplied by itself. Thus, $5^2 = 5 \times 5$ and $5^3 = 5 \times 5 \times 5$. The most often encountered exponent is 2, which is read as the *square* of a number. For example, 5^2 is read "five-squared."

Finding the *square root* of a number is the opposite procedure of squaring. The square root of a number, symbolized by the placement of a number under a radical sign ($\sqrt{\ }$), is that number which, when squared, will yield the number under the radical sign. Thus, $\sqrt{25} = 5$, $\sqrt{100} = 10$, and $\sqrt{27.04} = 5.2$. Although there is a long-hand method for deriving the square root of any number, the easiest method is to use an electronic calculator that has a square root key. If such a calculator is not available, then an alternative method is to use Table C.1, Appendix C.

Reference

Walker, Helen M. *Mathematics Essential for Elementary Statistics.* New York: Holt, Rinehart and Winston, 1951.

Solutions for Exercises

B

This appendix presents solutions for certain of the end-of-chapter exercises. It is not possible to give solutions for all exercises, because some allow students to develop individual solutions depending on their approach to the problem, while others involve evaluation of published research. Since such exercises have no single correct answer, it is recommended that they be discussed with fellow students and a course instructor.

Chapter 2
1a. Interval/ratio
 b. Nominal
 c. Interval/ratio
 d. Ordinal
 e. Nominal
2a. (a) Continuous
    (b) Discrete
    (c) Discrete
    (d) Continuous
    (e) Discrete
 b. (a) Standard unit
    (b) Qualitative classification/counting
    (c) Counting
    (d) Subjective ordinal ranking
    (e) Qualitative classification/counting
4a. 7, 13, 6, 28, 304, 10
 b. 7, 12, 6, 27, 304, 9
 c. 8, 13, 7, 28, 305, 10
5a. 0, 400, 1400
 b. 5.5, 420.2, 1360.0

Chapter 5
6. When the distribution is bimodal and emphasis is on the most typical observation. Also when a measure of central tendency is desired quickly.
7. When the distribution is markedly skewed.
8. $\overline{X}_w = 7.0$

Chapter 6
5a. Skewed positive, concentration at low end of range.
 b. Skewed negative, concentration at high end of range.
 c. Symmetrical, all three measures of central tendency at middle of range.
 d. Skewed negative, concentration at high end of range.
6. No, variation may be different. See Figure 5.2.

Chapter 7

	%Above	%Below
1a.	2.5	97.5
b.	97.5	2.5
c.	4.95	95.05
d.	95.05	4.95
e.	10.03	89.97
f.	89.97	10.03
g.	0.99	99.01
h.	99.01	0.99

4a. -1.50 (by definition)
 b. 118.2 mm Hg to 131.8 mm Hg *or* 13.6 mm Hg
 c. 98.58%
 d. 42.92%
 e. 42.92%
 f. 7.08%
 g. 7.08%

Chapter 8

1a. H_1: Structured preoperative teaching will significantly increase the adult surgical patient's ability to cough and deep-breathe as measured by vital capacity, maximum expiratory flow rate, and forced expiration volume.
H_2: Structured preoperative teaching will significantly reduce the average length of hospital stay for the adult surgical patient.
H_3: Structured preoperative teaching will significantly reduce the need for postoperative analgesics for the adult surgical patient.

 b. Directional

 c. Structured preoperative teaching will not significantly increase the adult surgical patient's ability to cough and deep-breathe as measured by vital capacity, maximum expiratory flow rate, and forced expiratory volume. Structured preoperative teaching will not significantly reduce average length of hospital stay for the adult surgical patient. Structured preoperative teaching will not significantly reduce the need for postoperative analgesics for the adult surgical patient.
NOTE: These hypotheses could also be stated in terms of predicting no differences between the two groups with regard to the variables under consideration.

 d. Reject the first and second, but accept the third *null* hypothesis. This means they are accepting the first and second, but rejecting the third *research* hypothesis.

 e. They are risking a type I error when they *reject* a null hypothesis and a type II error when they *accept* a null hypothesis.

 f. $p < .001$, since they report their findings as significant beyond the .001 level.

2a. Nurses differ in the amount of time they spend with dying and with non-dying patients.

b. Nurses communicate more (less) with dying than with non-dying patients.

c. There is no difference in the amount of time that nurses spend with dying and with non-dying patients.
There is no difference in the amount of verbal communication that nurses have with dying and non-dying patients.

d. Reject the null hypothesis.

e. Type I

f. There is no difference in the amount of verbal communication.

Chapter 10

1. Since these data are at the interval level, the median test makes better use of the information contained in the data than the chi-square test does.

2a. $U = 14$

b. H_1 : There is a significant difference between the satisfaction scores of the two groups.
$r = 10$

c. See discussion at the end of Chapter 10 comparing these two tests.

Chapter 11

1. Using a t test for independent samples of equal size, $t = 6.59$. In calculating this t value the data from the problem section of Chapter 3 were treated in terms of months or fractions thereof. Thus, 6 weeks was treated as 1.5 months, 7 weeks as 1.75 months, etc. An initiation of solid foods "at birth" or "immediately" was scored as zero in these calculations.

2. The t test is the most appropriate, since these are interval level data. However, the student may question whether the data meet all the assumptions underlying the t test. If they do not, then one of the other statistical tests would be more appropriate.

3. Using a t test for related samples, $t = 5.24$.

Chapter 12

1. $\lambda = .02$; no relationship.

2. $\gamma = .60; z = 3.47; p < .001$

$d_{yx} = .42; z = 4.00; p < .001$

$\tau_b = .42; z = 4.00; p < .001$

All three measures indicate a statistically significant positive relationship of moderate strength.

3. $\tau_c = -.66, z = -4.04; p < .001$

A statistically significant negative relationship which is moderately strong.

Chapter 13

2. $\hat{Y} = 107.2 - .6X$

3. $r = -.92$
   $r^2 = .85$

4. $t = -8.56; df = 13; p < .0005$

5. A statistically significant, strong negative relationship; age explains 85 percent of variation in percent RDA caloric intake.

6. $\hat{Y} = 91$

7. Decrease by 6 percent.

Statistical Tables

C

Table C.1. Squares and Square Roots of Integers from 1 to 1,000

Number	Square	Square Root	Number	Square	Square Root
1	1	1.000	41	16 81	6.403
2	4	1.414	42	17 64	6.481
3	9	1.732	43	18 49	6.557
4	16	2.000	44	19 36	6.633
5	25	2.236	45	20 25	6.708
6	36	2.449	46	21 16	6.782
7	49	2.646	47	22 09	6.856
8	64	2.828	48	23 04	6.928
9	81	3.000	49	24 01	7.000
10	1 00	3.162	50	25 00	7.071
11	1 21	3.317	51	26 01	7.141
12	1 44	3.464	52	27 04	7.211
13	1 69	3.606	53	28 09	7.280
14	1 96	3.742	54	29 16	7.348
15	2 25	3.873	55	30 25	7.416
16	2 56	4.000	56	31 36	7.483
17	2 89	4.123	57	32 49	7.550
18	3 24	4.243	58	33 64	7.616
19	3 61	4.359	59	34 81	7.681
20	4 00	4.472	60	36 00	7.746
21	4 41	4.583	61	37 21	7.810
22	4 84	4.690	62	38 44	7.874
23	5 29	4.796	63	39 69	7.937
24	5 76	4.899	64	40 96	8.000
25	6 25	5.000	65	42 25	8.062
26	6 76	5.099	66	43 56	8.124
27	7 29	5.196	67	44 89	8.185
28	7 84	5.292	68	46 24	8.246
29	8 41	5.385	69	47 61	8.307
30	9 00	5.477	70	49 00	8.367
31	9 61	5.568	71	50 41	8.426
32	10 24	5.657	72	51 84	8.485
33	10 89	5.745	73	53 29	8.544
34	11 56	5.831	74	54 76	8.602
35	12 25	5.916	75	56 25	8.660
36	12 96	6.000	76	57 76	8.718
37	13 69	6.083	77	59 29	8.775
38	14 44	6.164	78	60 84	8.832
39	15 21	6.245	79	62 41	8.888
40	16 00	6.325	80	64 00	8.944

Table C.1. (continued)

Number	Square	Square Root	Number	Square	Square Root
81	65 61	9.000	121	1 46 41	11.000
82	67 24	9.055	122	1 48 84	11.045
83	68 89	9.110	123	1 51 29	11.091
84	70 56	9.165	124	1 53 76	11.136
85	72 25	9.220	125	1 56 25	11.180
86	73 96	9.274	126	1 58 76	11.225
87	75 69	9.327	127	1 61 29	11.269
88	77 44	9.381	128	1 63 84	11.314
89	79 21	9.434	129	1 66 41	11.358
90	81 00	9.487	130	1 69 00	11.402
91	82 81	9.539	131	1 71 61	11.446
92	84 64	9.592	132	1 74 24	11.489
93	86 49	9.644	133	1 76 89	11.533
94	88 36	9.695	134	1 79 56	11.576
95	90 25	9.747	135	1 82 25	11.619
96	92 16	9.798	136	1 84 96	11.662
97	94 09	9.849	137	1 87 69	11.705
98	96 04	9.899	138	1 90 44	11.747
99	98 01	9.950	139	1 93 21	11.790
100	1 00 00	10.000	140	1 96 00	11.832
101	1 02 01	10.050	141	1 98 81	11.874
102	1 04 04	10.100	142	2 01 64	11.916
103	1 06 09	10.149	143	2 04 49	11.958
104	1 08 16	10.198	144	2 07 36	12.000
105	1 10 25	10.247	145	2 10 25	12.042
106	1 12 36	10.296	146	2 13 16	12.083
107	1 14 49	10.344	147	2 16 09	12.124
108	1 16 64	10.392	148	2 19 04	12.166
109	1 18 81	10.440	149	2 22 01	12.207
110	1 21 00	10.488	150	2 25 00	12.247
111	1 23 21	10.536	151	2 28 01	12.288
112	1 25 44	10.583	152	2 31 04	12.329
113	1 27 69	10.630	153	2 34 09	12.369
114	1 29 96	10.677	154	2 37 16	12.410
115	1 32 25	10.724	155	2 40 25	12.450
116	1 34 56	10.770	156	2 43 36	12.490
117	1 36 89	10.817	157	2 46 49	12.530
118	1 39 24	10.863	158	2 49 64	12.570
119	1 41 61	10.909	159	2 52 81	12.610
120	1 44 00	10.954	160	2 56 00	12.649

Table C.1. (continued)

Number	Square	Square Root	Number	Square	Square Root
161	2 59 21	12.689	201	4 04 01	14.177
162	2 62 44	12.728	202	4 08 04	14.213
163	2 65 69	12.767	203	4 12 09	14.248
164	2 68 96	12.806	204	4 16 16	14.283
165	2 72 25	12.845	205	4 20 25	14.318
166	2 75 56	12.884	206	4 24 36	14.353
167	2 78 89	12.923	207	4 28 49	14.387
168	2 82 24	12.961	208	4 32 64	14.422
169	2 85 61	13.000	209	4 36 81	14.457
170	2 89 00	13.038	210	4 41 00	14.491
171	2 92 41	13.077	211	4 45 21	14.526
172	2 95 84	13.115	212	4 49 44	14.560
173	2 99 29	13.153	213	4 53 69	14.595
174	3 02 76	13.191	214	4 57 96	14.629
175	3 06 25	13.229	215	4 62 25	14.663
176	3 09 76	13.266	216	4 66 56	14.697
177	3 13 29	13.304	217	4 70 89	14.731
178	3 16 84	13.342	218	4 75 24	14.765
179	3 20 41	13.379	219	4 79 61	14.799
180	3 24 00	13.416	220	4 84 00	14.832
181	3 27 61	13.454	221	4 88 41	14.866
182	3 31 24	13.491	222	4 92 84	14.900
183	3 34 89	13.528	223	4 97 29	14.933
184	3 38 56	13.565	224	5 01 76	14.967
185	3 42 25	13.601	225	5 06 25	15.000
186	3 45 96	13.638	226	5 10 76	15.033
187	3 49 69	13.675	227	5 15 29	15.067
188	3 53 44	13.711	228	5 19 84	15.100
189	3 57 21	13.748	229	5 24 41	15.133
190	3 61 00	13.784	230	5 29 00	15.166
191	3 64 81	13.820	231	5 33 61	15.199
192	3 68 64	13.856	232	5 38 24	15.232
193	3 72 49	13.892	233	5 42 89	15.264
194	3 76 36	13.928	234	5 47 56	15.297
195	3 80 25	13.964	235	5 52 25	15.330
196	3 84 16	14.000	236	5 56 96	15.362
197	3 88 09	14.036	237	5 61 69	15.395
198	3 92 04	14.071	238	5 66 44	15.427
199	3 96 01	14.107	239	5 71 21	15.460
200	4 00 00	14.142	240	5 76 00	15.492

Table C.1. (continued)

Number	Square	Square Root	Number	Square	Square Root
241	5 80 81	15.524	281	7 89 61	16.763
242	5 85 64	15.556	282	7 95 24	16.793
243	5 90 49	15.588	283	8 00 89	16.823
244	5 95 36	15.620	284	8 06 56	16.852
245	6 00 25	15.652	285	8 12 25	16.882
246	6 05 16	15.684	286	8 17 96	16.912
247	6 10 09	15.716	287	8 23 69	16.941
248	6 15 04	15.748	288	8 29 44	16.971
249	6 20 01	15.780	289	8 35 21	17.000
250	6 25 00	15.811	290	8 41 00	17.029
251	6 30 01	15.843	291	8 46 81	17.059
252	6 35 04	15.875	292	8 52 64	17.088
253	6 40 09	15.906	293	8 58 49	17.117
254	6 45 16	15.937	294	8 64 36	17.146
255	6 50 25	15.969	295	8 70 25	17.176
256	6 55 36	16.000	296	8 76 16	17.205
257	6 60 49	16.031	297	8 82 09	17.234
258	6 65 64	16.062	298	8 88 04	17.263
259	6 70 81	16.093	299	8 94 01	17.292
260	6 76 00	16.125	300	9 00 00	17.321
261	6 81 21	16.155	301	9 06 01	17.349
262	6 86 44	16.186	302	9 12 04	17.378
263	6 91 69	16.217	303	9 18 09	17.407
264	6 96 96	16.248	304	9 24 16	17.436
265	7 02 25	16.279	305	9 30 25	17.464
266	7 07 56	16.310	306	9 36 36	17.493
267	7 12 89	16.340	307	9 42 49	17.521
268	7 18 24	16.371	308	9 48 64	17.550
269	7 23 61	16.401	309	9 54 81	17.578
270	7 29 00	16.432	310	9 61 00	17.607
271	7 34 41	16.462	311	9 67 21	17.635
272	7 39 84	16.492	312	9 73 44	17.664
273	7 45 29	16.523	313	9 79 69	17.692
274	7 50 76	16.553	314	9 85 96	17.720
275	7 56 25	16.583	315	9 92 25	17.748
276	7 61 76	16.613	316	9 98 56	17.776
277	7 67 29	16.643	317	10 04 89	17.804
278	7 72 84	16.673	318	10 11 24	17.833
279	7 78 41	16.703	319	10 17 61	17.861
280	7 84 00	16.733	320	10 24 00	17.889

Table C.1. (continued)

Number	Square	Square Root	Number	Square	Square Root
321	10 30 41	17.916	361	13 03 21	19.000
322	10 36 84	17.944	362	13 10 44	19.026
323	10 43 29	17.972	363	13 17 69	19.053
324	10 49 76	18.000	364	13 24 96	19.079
325	10 56 25	18.028	365	13 32 25	19.105
326	10 62 76	18.055	366	13 39 56	19.131
327	10 69 29	18.083	367	13 46 89	19.157
328	10 75 84	18.111	368	13 54 24	19.183
329	10 82 41	18.138	369	13 61 61	19.209
330	10 89 00	18.166	370	13 69 00	19.235
331	10 95 61	18.193	371	13 76 41	19.261
332	11 02 24	18.221	372	13 83 84	19.287
333	11 08 89	18.248	373	13 91 29	19.313
334	11 15 56	18.276	374	13 98 76	19.339
335	11 22 25	18.303	375	14 06 25	19.363
336	11 28 96	18.330	376	14 13 76	19.391
337	11 35 69	18.358	377	14 21 29	19.416
338	11 42 44	18.385	378	14 28 84	19.442
339	11 49 21	18.412	379	14 36 41	19.468
340	11 56 00	18.439	380	14 44 00	19.494
341	11 62 81	18.466	381	14 51 61	19.519
342	11 69 64	18.493	382	14 59 24	19.545
343	11 76 49	18.520	383	14 66 89	19.570
344	11 83 36	18.547	384	14 74 56	19.596
345	11 90 25	18.574	385	14 82 25	19.621
346	11 97 16	18.601	386	14 89 96	19.647
347	12 04 09	18.628	387	14 97 69	19.672
348	12 11 04	18.655	388	15 05 44	19.698
349	12 18 01	18.682	389	15 13 21	19.723
350	12 25 00	18.708	390	15 21 00	19.748
351	12 32 01	18.735	391	15 28 81	19.774
352	12 39 04	18.762	392	15 36 64	19.799
353	12 46 09	18.788	393	15 44 49	19.824
354	12 53 16	18.815	394	15 52 36	19.849
355	12 60 25	18.841	395	15 60 25	19.875
356	12 67 36	18.868	396	15 68 16	19.900
357	12 74 49	18.894	397	15 76 09	19.925
358	12 81 64	18.921	398	15 84 04	19.950
359	12 88 81	18.947	399	15 92 01	19.975
360	12 96 00	18.974	400	16 00 00	20.000

Table C.1. (continued)

Number	Square	Square Root	Number	Square	Square Root
401	16 08 01	20.025	441	19 44 81	21.000
402	16 16 04	20.050	442	19 53 64	21.024
403	16 24 09	20.075	443	19 62 49	21.048
404	16 32 16	20.100	444	19 71 36	21.071
405	16 40 25	20.125	445	19 80 25	21.095
406	16 48 36	20.149	446	19 89 16	21.119
407	16 56 49	20.174	447	19 98 09	21.142
408	16 64 64	20.199	448	20 07 04	21.166
409	16 72 81	20.224	449	20 16 01	21.190
410	16 81 00	20.248	450	20 25 00	21.213
411	16 89 21	20.273	451	20 34 01	21.237
412	16 97 44	20.298	452	20 43 04	21.260
413	17 05 69	20.322	453	20 52 09	21.284
414	17 13 96	20.347	454	20 61 16	21.307
415	17 22 25	20.372	455	20 70 25	21.331
416	17 30 56	20.396	456	20 79 36	21.354
417	17 38 89	20.421	457	20 88 49	21.378
418	17 47 24	20.445	458	20 97 64	21.401
419	17 55 61	20.469	459	21 06 81	21.424
420	17 64 00	20.494	460	21 16 00	21.448
421	17 72 41	20.518	461	21 25 21	21.471
422	17 80 84	20.543	462	21 34 44	21.494
423	17 89 29	20.567	463	21 43 69	21.517
424	17 97 76	20.591	464	21 52 96	21.541
425	18 06 25	20.616	465	21 62 25	21.564
426	18 14 76	20.640	466	21 71 56	21.587
427	18 23 29	20.664	467	21 80 89	21.610
428	18 31 84	20.688	468	21 90 24	21.633
429	18 40 41	20.712	469	21 99 61	21.656
430	18 49 00	20.736	470	22 09 00	21.679
431	18 57 61	20.761	471	22 18 41	21.703
432	18 66 24	20.785	472	22 27 84	21.726
433	18 74 89	20.809	473	22 37 29	21.749
434	18 83 56	20.833	474	22 46 76	21.772
435	18 92 25	20.857	475	22 56 25	21.794
436	19 00 96	20.881	476	22 65 76	21.817
437	19 09 69	20.905	477	22 75 29	21.840
438	19 18 44	20.928	478	22 84 84	21.863
439	19 27 21	20.952	479	22 94 41	21.886
440	19 36 00	20.976	480	23 04 00	21.909

Table C.1. (continued)

Number	Square	Square Root	Number	Square	Square Root
481	23 13 61	21.932	521	27 14 41	22.825
482	23 23 24	21.954	522	27 24 84	22.847
483	23 32 89	21.977	523	27 35 29	22.869
484	23 42 56	22.000	524	27 45 76	22.891
485	23 52 25	22.023	525	27 56 25	22.913
486	23 61 96	22.045	526	27 66 76	22.935
487	23 71 69	22.068	527	27 77 29	22.956
488	23 81 44	22.091	528	27 87 84	22.978
489	23 91 21	22.113	529	27 98 41	23.000
490	24 01 00	22.136	530	28 09 00	23.022
491	24 10 81	22.159	531	28 19 61	23.043
492	24 20 64	22.181	532	28 30 24	23.065
493	24 30 49	22.204	533	28 40 89	23.087
494	24 40 36	22.226	534	28 51 56	23.108
495	24 50 25	22.249	535	28 62 25	23.130
496	24 60 16	22.271	536	28 72 96	23.152
497	24 70 09	22.293	537	28 83 69	23.173
498	24 80 04	22.316	538	28 94 44	23.195
499	24 90 01	22.338	539	29 05 21	23.216
500	25 00 00	22.361	540	29 16 00	23.238
501	25 10 01	22.383	541	29 26 81	23.259
502	25 20 04	22.405	542	29 37 64	23.281
503	25 30 09	22.428	543	29 48 49	23.302
504	25 40 16	22.450	544	29 59 36	23.324
505	25 50 25	22.472	545	29 70 25	23.345
506	25 60 36	22.494	546	29 81 16	23.367
507	25 70 49	22.517	547	29 92 09	23.388
508	25 80 64	22.539	548	30 03 04	23.409
509	25 90 81	22.561	549	30 14 01	23.431
510	26 01 00	22.583	550	30 25 00	23.452
511	26 11 21	22.605	551	30 36 01	23.473
512	26 21 44	22.627	552	30 47 04	23.495
513	26 31 69	22.650	553	30 58 09	23.516
514	26 41 96	22.672	554	30 69 16	23.537
515	26 52 25	22.694	555	30 80 25	23.558
516	26 62 56	22.716	556	30 91 36	23.580
517	26 72 89	22.738	557	31 02 49	23.601
518	26 83 24	22.760	558	31 13 64	23.622
519	26 93 61	22.782	559	31 24 81	23.643
520	27 04 00	22.804	560	31 36 00	23.664

Table C.1. (continued)

Number	Square	Square Root	Number	Square	Square Root
561	31 47 21	23.685	601	36 12 01	24.515
562	31 58 44	23.707	602	36 24 04	24.536
563	31 69 69	23.728	603	36 36 09	24.556
564	31 80 96	23.749	604	36 48 16	24.576
565	31 92 25	23.770	605	36 60 25	24.597
566	32 03 56	23.791	606	36 72 36	24.617
567	32 14 89	23.812	607	36 84 49	24.637
568	32 26 24	23.833	608	36 96 64	24.658
569	32 37 61	23.854	609	37 08 81	24.678
570	32 49 00	23.875	610	37 21 00	24.698
571	32 60 41	23.896	611	37 33 21	24.718
572	32 71 84	23.917	612	37 45 44	24.739
573	32 83 29	23.937	613	37 57 69	24.759
574	32 94 76	23.958	614	37 69 96	24.779
575	33 06 25	23.979	615	37 82 25	24.799
576	33 17 76	24.000	616	37 94 56	24.819
577	33 29 29	24.021	617	38 06 89	24.839
578	33 40 84	24.042	618	38 19 24	24.860
579	33 52 41	24.062	619	38 31 61	24.880
580	33 64 00	24.083	620	38 44 00	24.900
581	33 75 61	24.104	621	38 56 41	24.920
582	33 87 24	24.125	622	38 68 84	24.940
583	33 98 89	24.145	623	38 81 29	24.960
584	34 10 56	24.166	624	38 93 76	24.980
585	34 22 25	24.187	625	39 06 25	25.000
586	34 33 96	24.207	626	39 18 76	25.020
587	34 45 69	24.228	627	39 31 29	25.040
588	34 57 44	24.249	628	39 43 84	25.060
589	34 69 21	24.269	629	39 56 41	25.080
590	34 81 00	24.290	630	39 69 00	25.100
591	34 92 81	24.310	631	39 81 61	25.120
592	35 04 64	24.331	632	39 94 24	25.140
593	35 16 49	24.352	633	40 06 89	25.159
594	35 28 36	24.372	634	40 19 56	25.179
595	35 40 25	24.393	635	40 32 25	25.199
596	35 52 16	24.413	636	40 44 96	25.219
597	35 64 09	24.434	637	40 57 69	25.239
598	35 76 04	24.454	638	40 70 44	25.259
599	35 88 01	24.474	639	40 83 21	25.278
600	36 00 00	24.495	640	40 96 00	25.298

Table C.1. (continued)

Number	Square	Square Root	Number	Square	Square Root
641	41 08 81	25.318	681	46 37 61	26.096
642	41 21 64	25.338	682	46 51 24	26.115
643	41 34 49	25.357	683	46 64 89	26.134
644	41 47 36	25.377	684	46 78 56	26.153
645	41 60 25	25.397	685	46 92 25	26.173
646	41 73 16	25.417	686	47 05 96	26.192
647	41 86 09	25.436	687	47 19 69	26.211
648	41 99 04	25.456	688	47 33 44	26.230
649	42 12 01	25.475	689	47 47 21	26.249
650	42 25 00	25.495	690	47 61 00	26.268
651	42 38 01	25.515	691	47 74 81	26.287
652	42 51 04	25.534	692	47 88 64	26.306
653	42 64 09	25.554	693	48 02 49	26.325
654	42 77 16	25.573	694	48 16 36	26.344
655	42 90 25	25.593	695	48 30 25	26.363
656	43 03 36	25.612	696	48 44 16	26.382
657	43 16 49	25.632	697	48 58 09	26.401
658	43 29 64	25.652	698	48 72 04	26.420
659	43 42 81	25.671	699	48 86 01	26.439
660	43 56 00	25.690	700	49 00 00	26.458
661	43 69 21	25.710	701	49 14 01	26.476
662	43 82 44	25.729	702	49 28 04	26.495
663	43 95 69	25.749	703	49 42 09	26.514
664	44 08 96	25.768	704	49 56 16	26.533
665	44 22 25	25.788	705	49 70 25	26.552
666	44 35 56	25.807	706	49 84 36	26.571
667	44 48 89	25.826	707	49 98 49	26.589
668	44 62 24	25.846	708	50 12 64	26.608
669	44 75 61	25.865	709	50 26 81	26.627
670	44 89 00	25.884	710	50 41 00	26.646
671	45 02 41	25.904	711	50 55 21	26.665
672	45 15 84	25.923	712	50 69 44	26.683
673	45 29 29	25.942	713	50 83 69	26.702
674	45 42 76	25.962	714	50 97 96	26.721
675	45 56 25	25.981	715	51 12 25	26.739
676	45 69 76	26.000	716	51 26 56	26.758
677	45 83 29	26.019	717	51 40 89	26.777
678	45 96 84	26.038	718	51 55 24	26.796
679	46 10 41	26.058	719	51 69 61	26.814
680	46 24 00	26.077	720	51 84 00	26.833

Table C.1. (continued)

Number	Square	Square Root	Number	Square	Square Root
721	51 98 41	26.851	761	57 91 21	27.586
722	52 12 84	26.870	762	58 06 44	27.604
723	52 27 29	26.889	763	58 21 69	27.622
724	52 41 76	26.907	764	58 36 96	27.641
725	52 56 25	26.926	765	58 52 25	27.659
726	52 70 76	26.944	766	58 67 56	27.677
727	52 85 29	26.963	767	58 82 89	27.695
728	52 99 84	26.981	768	58 98 24	27.713
729	53 14 41	27.000	769	59 13 61	27.731
730	53 29 00	27.019	770	59 29 00	27.749
731	53 43 61	27.037	771	59 44 41	27.767
732	53 58 24	27.055	772	59 59 84	27.785
733	53 72 89	27.074	773	59 75 29	27.803
734	53 87 56	27.092	774	59 90 76	27.821
735	54 02 25	27.111	775	60 06 25	27.839
736	54 16 96	27.129	776	60 21 76	27.857
737	54 31 69	27.148	777	60 37 29	27.875
738	54 46 44	27.166	778	60 52 84	27.893
739	54 61 21	27.185	779	60 68 41	27.911
740	54 76 00	27.203	780	60 84 00	27.928
741	54 90 81	27.221	781	60 99 61	27.946
742	55 05 64	27.240	782	61 15 24	27.964
743	55 20 49	27.258	783	61 30 89	27.982
744	55 35 36	27.276	784	61 46 56	28.000
745	55 50 25	27.295	785	61 62 25	28.018
746	55 65 16	27.313	786	61 77 96	28.036
747	55 80 09	27.331	787	61 93 69	28.054
748	55 95 04	27.350	788	62 09 44	28.071
749	56 10 01	27.368	789	62 25 21	28.089
750	56 25 00	27.386	790	62 41 00	28.107
751	56 40 01	27.404	791	62 56 81	28.125
752	56 55 04	27.423	792	62 72 64	28.142
753	56 70 09	27.441	793	62 88 49	28.160
754	56 85 16	27.459	794	63 04 36	28.178
755	57 00 25	27.477	795	63 20 25	28.196
756	57 15 36	27.495	796	63 36 16	28.213
757	57 30 49	27.514	797	63 52 09	28.231
758	57 45 64	27.532	798	63 68 04	28.249
759	57 60 81	27.550	799	63 84 01	28.267
760	57 76 00	27.568	800	64 00 00	28.284

Table C.1. (continued)

Number	Square	Square Root	Number	Square	Square Root
801	64 16 01	28.302	841	70 72 81	29.000
802	64 32 04	28.320	842	70 89 64	29.017
803	64 48 09	28.337	843	71 06 49	29.034
804	64 64 16	28.355	844	71 23 36	29.052
805	64 80 25	28.373	845	71 40 25	29.069
806	64 96 36	28.390	846	71 57 16	29.086
807	65 12 49	28.408	847	71 74 09	29.103
808	65 28 64	28.425	848	71 91 04	29.120
809	65 44 81	28.443	849	72 08 01	29.138
810	65 61 00	28.460	850	72 25 00	29.155
811	65 77 21	28.478	851	72 42 01	29.172
812	65 93 44	28.496	852	72 59 04	29.189
813	66 09 69	28.513	853	72 76 09	29.206
814	66 25 96	28.531	854	72 93 16	29.223
815	66 42 25	28.548	855	73 10 25	29.240
816	66 58 56	28.566	856	73 27 36	29.257
817	66 74 89	28.583	857	73 44 49	29.275
818	66 91 24	28.601	858	73 61 64	29.292
819	67 07 61	28.618	859	73 78 81	29.309
820	67 24 00	28.636	860	73 96 00	29.326
821	67 40 41	28.653	861	74 13 21	29.343
822	67 56 84	28.671	862	74 30 44	29.360
823	67 73 29	28.688	863	74 47 69	29.377
824	67 89 76	28.705	864	74 64 96	29.394
825	68 06 25	28.723	865	74 82 25	29.411
826	68 22 76	28.740	866	74 99 56	29.428
827	68 39 29	28.758	867	75 16 89	29.445
828	68 55 84	28.775	868	75 34 24	29.462
829	68 72 41	28.792	869	75 51 61	29.479
830	68 89 00	28.810	870	75 69 00	29.496
831	69 05 61	28.827	871	75 86 41	29.513
832	69 22 24	28.844	872	76 03 84	29.530
833	69 38 89	28.862	873	76 21 29	29.547
834	69 55 56	28.879	874	76 38 76	29.563
835	69 72 25	28.896	875	76 56 25	29.580
836	69 88 96	28.914	876	76 73 76	29.597
837	70 05 69	28.931	877	76 91 29	29.614
838	70 22 44	28.948	878	77 08 84	29.631
839	70 39 21	28.965	879	77 26 41	29.648
840	70 56 00	28.983	880	77 44 00	29.665

Table C.1. (continued)

Number	Square	Square Root	Number	Square	Square Root
881	77 61 61	29.682	921	84 82 41	30.348
882	77 79 24	29.698	922	85 00 84	30.364
883	77 96 89	29.715	923	85 19 29	30.381
884	78 14 56	29.732	924	85 37 76	30.397
885	78 32 25	29.749	925	85 56 25	30.414
886	78 49 96	29.766	926	85 74 76	30.430
887	78 67 69	29.783	927	85 93 29	30.447
888	78 85 44	29.799	928	86 11 84	30.463
889	79 03 21	29.816	929	86 30 41	30.480
890	79 21 00	29.833	930	86 49 00	30.496
891	79 38 81	29.850	931	86 67 61	30.512
892	79 56 64	29.866	932	86 86 24	30.529
893	79 74 49	29.883	933	87 04 89	30.545
894	79 92 36	29.900	934	87 23 56	30.561
895	80 10 25	29.916	935	87 42 25	30.578
896	80 28 16	29.933	936	87 60 96	30.594
897	80 46 09	29.950	937	87 79 69	30.610
898	80 64 04	29.967	938	87 98 44	30.627
899	80 82 01	29.983	939	88 17 21	30.643
900	81 00 00	30.000	940	88 36 00	30.659
901	81 80 01	30.017	941	88 54 81	30.676
902	81 36 04	30.033	942	88 73 64	30.692
903	81 54 09	30.050	943	88 92 49	30.708
904	81 72 16	30.067	944	89 11 36	30.725
905	81 90 25	30.083	945	89 30 25	30.741
906	82 08 36	30.100	946	89 49 16	30.757
907	82 26 49	30.116	947	89 68 09	30.773
908	82 44 64	30.133	948	89 87 04	30.790
909	82 62 81	30.150	949	90 06 01	30.806
910	82 81 00	30.166	950	90 25 00	30.822
911	82 99 21	30.183	951	90 44 01	30.838
912	83 17 44	30.199	952	90 63 04	30.854
913	83 35 69	30.216	953	90 82 09	30.871
914	83 53 96	30.232	954	91 01 16	30.887
915	83 72 25	30.249	955	91 20 25	30.903
916	83 90 56	30.265	956	91 39 36	30.919
917	84 08 89	30.282	957	91 58 49	30.935
918	84 27 24	30.299	958	91 77 64	30.952
919	84 45 61	30.315	959	91 96 81	30.968
920	84 64 00	30.332	960	92 16 00	30.984

Table C.1. (continued)

Number	Square	Square Root	Number	Square	Square Root
961	92 35 21	31.000	981	96 23 61	31.321
962	92 54 44	31.016	982	96 43 24	31.337
963	92 73 69	31.032	983	96 62 89	31.353
964	92 92 96	31.048	984	96 82 56	31.369
965	93 12 25	31.064	985	97 02 25	31.385
966	93 31 56	31.081	986	97 21 96	31.401
967	93 50 89	31.097	987	97 41 69	31.417
968	93 70 24	31.113	988	97 61 44	31.432
969	93 89 61	31.129	989	97 81 21	31.448
970	94 09 00	31.145	990	98 01 00	31.464
971	94 28 41	31.161	991	98 20 81	31.480
972	94 47 84	31.177	992	98 40 64	31.496
973	94 67 29	31.193	993	98 60 49	31.512
974	94 86 76	31.209	994	98 80 36	31.528
975	95 06 25	31.225	995	99 00 25	31.544
976	95 25 76	31.241	996	99 20 16	31.559
977	95 45 29	31.257	997	99 40 09	31.575
978	95 64 84	31.273	998	99 60 04	31.591
979	95 84 41	31.289	999	99 80 01	31.607
980	96 04 00	31.305	1000	100 00 00	31.623

Source: John A. Mueller, Karl F. Schuessler, and Herbert L. Costner, *Statistical Reasoning in Sociology*, 1977. Reprinted with permission of the authors and Houghton Mifflin Company.

How To Use Table C.2

The proportion of the normal distribution located beyond a given z score is presented in the body of Table C.2, while the corresponding z score is listed in the left and top margins. The first two digits of the z score value are listed in the left margin, and the third digit is listed in the top margin. Because the normal distribution is perfectly symmetrical, only positive z score values are presented. The proportions apply equally to positive and negative z score values.

FINDING THE PROPORTION BEYOND A POSITIVE Z SCORE
If $z = +1.65$, locate 1.6 in the left margin and 5 in the top margin. The proportion listed at the intersection of this row and column is .0495.

FINDING THE PROPORTION BEYOND A NEGATIVE Z SCORE
If $z = -1.65$, follow the same procedure as for $z = +1.65$. Note that although the proportion is identical for both z score values, they have opposite locations: the plus value occupies a right-hand portion of the normal distribution curve, whereas the minus value occupies a left-hand portion.

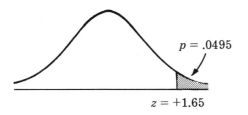
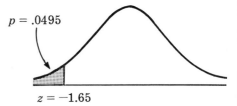

$p = .0495$

$p = .0495$

$z = +1.65$ $z = -1.65$

Z-Score Values for Frequently Used Significance Levels (α)

α	One-tailed test	Two-tailed test
.10	1.28	1.65
.05	1.65	1.96
.01	2.33	2.58
.001	3.09	3.30

Table C.2. Proportions of the Normal Distribution Beyond a Given z-Score

z	0	1	2	3	4	5	6	7	8	9
0.0	.5000	.4960	.4920	.4880	.4840	.4801	.4761	.4721	.4681	.4641
0.1	.4602	.4562	.4522	.4483	.4443	.4404	.4364	.4325	.4286	.4247
0.2	.4207	.4168	.4129	.4090	.4052	.4013	.3974	.3936	.3897	.3859
0.3	.3821	.3783	.3745	.3707	.3669	.3632	.3594	.3557	.3520	.3483
0.4	.3446	.3409	.3372	.3336	.3300	.3264	.3228	.3192	.3156	.3121
0.5	.3085	.3050	.3015	.2981	.2946	.2912	.2877	.2843	.2810	.2776
0.6	.2743	.2709	.2676	.2643	.2611	.2578	.2546	.2514	.2483	.2451
0.7	.2420	.2389	.2358	.2327	.2296	.2266	.2236	.2206	.2177	.2148
0.8	.2119	.2090	.2061	.2033	.2005	.1977	.1949	.1922	.1894	.1867
0.9	.1841	.1814	.1788	.1762	.1736	.1711	.1685	.1660	.1635	.1611
1.0	.1587	.1562	.1539	.1515	.1492	.1469	.1446	.1423	.1401	.1379
1.1	.1357	.1335	.1314	.1292	.1271	.1251	.1230	.1210	.1190	.1170
1.2	.1151	.1131	.1112	.1093	.1075	.1056	.1038	.1020	.1003	.0985
1.3	.0968	.0951	.0934	.0918	.0901	.0885	.0869	.0853	.0838	.0823
1.4	.0808	.0793	.0778	.0764	.0749	.0735	.0721	.0708	.0694	.0681
1.5	.0668	.0655	.0643	.0630	.0618	.0606	.0594	.0582	.0571	.0559
1.6	.0548	.0537	.0526	.0516	.0505	.0495	.0485	.0475	.0465	.0455
1.7	.0446	.0436	.0427	.0418	.0409	.0401	.0392	.0384	.0375	.0367
1.8	.0359	.0351	.0344	.0336	.0329	.0322	.0314	.0307	.0301	.0294
1.9	.0287	.0281	.0274	.0268	.0262	.0256	.0250	.0244	.0239	.0233
2.0	.0228	.0222	.0217	.0212	.0207	.0202	.0197	.0192	.0188	.0183
2.1	.0179	.0174	.0170	.0166	.0162	.0158	.0154	.0150	.0146	.0143
2.2	.0139	.0136	.0132	.0129	.0125	.0122	.0119	.0116	.0113	.0110
2.3	.0107	.0104	.0102	.0099	.0096	.0094	.0091	.0089	.0087	.0084
2.4	.0082	.0080	.0078	.0075	.0073	.0071	.0069	.0068	.0066	.0064
2.5	.0062	.0060	.0059	.0057	.0055	.0054	.0052	.0051	.0049	.0048
2.6	.0047	.0045	.0044	.0043	.0041	.0040	.0039	.0038	.0037	.0036
2.7	.0035	.0034	.0033	.0032	.0031	.0030	.0029	.0028	.0027	.0026
2.8	.0026	.0025	.0024	.0023	.0023	.0022	.0021	.0021	.0020	.0019
2.9	.0019	.0018	.0018	.0017	.0016	.0016	.0015	.0015	.0014	.0014
3.0	.0013	.0013	.0013	.0012	.0012	.0011	.0011	.0011	.0010	.0010

Source: As adapted from Wallis and Roberts, *Statistics, A New Approach*, 1956, by Theodore R. Anderson and Morris Zelditch, Jr., *A Basic Course in Statistics with Sociological Applications*, 1975. Reprinted with permission of the authors, the Macmillan Company, and Holt, Rinehart and Winston, Inc.

Table C.3. Minimum Values of Chi-Square to Reject H_0.

df	$P = .30$	.20	.10	.05	.02	.01	.001
1	1.074	1.642	2.706	3.841	5.412	6.635	10.827
2	2.408	3.219	4.605	5.991	7.824	9.210	13.815
3	3.665	4.642	6.251	7.815	9.837	11.345	16.268
4	4.878	5.989	7.779	9.488	11.668	13.277	18.465
5	6.064	7.289	9.236	11.070	13.388	15.086	20.517
6	7.231	8.558	10.645	12.592	15.033	16.812	22.457
7	8.383	9.803	12.017	14.067	16.622	18.475	24.322
8	9.524	11.030	13.362	15.507	18.168	20.090	26.125
9	10.656	12.242	14.684	16.919	19.679	21.666	27.877
10	11.781	13.442	15.987	18.307	21.161	23.209	29.588
11	12.899	14.631	17.275	19.675	22.618	24.725	31.264
12	14.011	15.812	18.549	21.026	24.054	26.217	32.909
13	15.119	16.985	19.812	22.362	25.472	27.688	34.528
14	16.222	18.151	21.064	23.685	26.873	29.141	36.123
15	17.322	19.311	22.307	24.996	28.259	30.578	37.697
16	18.418	20.465	23.542	26.296	29.633	32.000	39.252
17	19.511	21.615	24.769	27.587	30.995	33.409	40.790
18	20.601	22.760	25.989	28.869	32.346	34.805	42.312
19	21.689	23.900	27.204	30.144	33.687	36.191	43.820
20	22.775	25.038	28.412	31.410	35.020	37.566	45.315
21	23.858	26.171	29.615	32.671	36.343	38.932	46.797
22	24.939	27.301	30.813	33.924	37.659	40.289	48.268
23	26.018	28.429	32.007	35.172	38.968	41.638	49.728
24	27.096	29.553	33.196	36.415	40.270	42.980	51.179
25	28.172	30.675	34.382	37.652	41.566	44.314	52.620
26	29.246	31.795	35.563	38.885	42.856	45.642	54.052
27	30.319	32.912	36.741	40.113	44.140	46.963	55.476
28	31.391	34.027	37.916	41.337	45.419	48.278	56.893
29	32.461	35.139	39.087	42.557	46.693	49.588	58.302
30	33.530	36.250	40.256	43.773	47.962	50.892	59.703

Source: Adapted from Fisher and Yates, *Statistical Tables for Biological, Agricultural and Medical Research*, 1948, published by Longman Group Ltd., London (previously published by Oliver & Boyd, Edinburgh), with permission of the authors and publishers.

How to Use Table C.3

Locate degrees of freedom (df) in the left margin and level of significance in the top margin. The minimum chi-square value required to reject H_0 is listed at the intersection of that row and column. When df > 30, chi-square may be converted into a z score by the formula $z = \sqrt{2 \chi^2} - \sqrt{2df - 1}$, remembering that the probability of chi-square corresponds to that of a single tail of the normal curve shown in Table C.2.

Example

df = 6

$\alpha = .05$

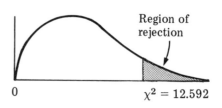

Region of rejection

0

$\chi^2 = 12.592$

How to Use Table C.4

If this table is used, the value of n_1 must be between 1 and 20. The value of n_2 must be between 9 and 20. Select the appropriate subtable, a, b, or c, depending on level of significance and whether a one- or two-tailed test is being applied. Specific subtables apply to the following situations:

C.4a: One-tailed test when $\alpha = .01$
Two-tailed test when $\alpha = .02$

C.4b: One-tailed test when $\alpha = .025$
Two-tailed test when $\alpha = .05$

C.4c: One-tailed test when $\alpha = .05$
Two-tailed test when $\alpha = .10$

Locate the n_2 value of interest among the values listed across the top of the table. Locate the n_1 value of interest among the values listed in the stub column (far left) of the table. Locate the intersection of the n_2 column and the n_1 row in the body of the table. Compare this table value with the calculated U value. If the calculated U value is *less or equal* to the table value, *reject H_0*. If the calculated U is *greater* than the table value, *accept H_0*.

Example 1

H_1: Nondirectional
α: .05
$n_1 = 13, n_2 = 15$
$U = 50$

Inference Decision

(Use Table C.4b)
Reject H_0, since U value of 50 is *smaller* than table value of 54.

Example 2

H_1: Directional
α: .01
$n_1 = 9, n_2 = 11$
$U = 20$

Inference Decision

(Use Table C.4a)
Accept H_0, since U value of 20 is *greater* than table value of 18.

Example 3

H_1: Directional
α: .05
$n_1 = 12, n_2 = 9$
$U = 30$

Inference Decision

(Use Table C.4c)
Reject H_0, since U value of 30 is *equal* to table value of 30.

Table C.4. Maximum Values of U in the Mann-Whitney Test to Reject H_0.

a. One-tailed test when $\alpha = .01$; two-tailed test when $\alpha = .02$

N_2 / N_1	9	10	11	12	13	14	15	16	17	18	19	20
1												
2					0	0	0	0	0	0	1	1
3	1	1	1	2	2	2	3	3	4	4	4	5
4	3	3	4	5	5	6	7	7	8	9	9	10
5	5	6	7	8	9	10	11	12	13	14	15	16
6	7	8	9	11	12	13	15	16	18	19	20	22
7	9	11	12	14	16	17	19	21	23	24	26	28
8	11	13	15	17	20	22	24	26	28	30	32	34
9	14	16	18	21	23	26	28	31	33	36	38	40
10	16	19	22	24	27	30	33	36	38	41	44	47
11	18	22	25	28	31	34	37	41	44	47	50	53
12	21	24	28	31	35	38	42	46	49	53	56	60
13	23	27	31	35	39	43	47	51	55	59	63	67
14	26	30	34	38	43	47	51	56	60	65	69	73
15	28	33	37	42	47	51	56	61	66	70	75	80
16	31	36	41	46	51	56	61	66	71	76	82	87
17	33	38	44	49	55	60	66	71	77	82	88	93
18	36	41	47	53	59	65	70	76	82	88	94	100
19	38	44	50	56	63	69	75	82	88	94	101	107
20	40	47	53	60	67	73	80	87	93	100	107	114

b. One-tailed test when $\alpha = .025$; two-tailed test when $\alpha = .05$

N_2 / N_1	9	10	11	12	13	14	15	16	17	18	19	20
1												
2	0	0	0	1	1	1	1	1	2	2	2	2
3	2	3	3	4	4	5	5	6	6	7	7	8
4	4	5	6	7	8	9	10	11	11	12	13	13
5	7	8	9	11	12	13	14	15	17	18	19	20
6	10	11	13	14	16	17	19	21	22	24	25	27
7	12	14	16	18	20	22	24	26	28	30	32	34
8	15	17	19	22	24	26	29	31	34	36	38	41
9	17	20	23	26	28	31	34	37	39	42	45	48
10	20	23	26	29	33	36	39	42	45	48	52	55
11	23	26	30	33	37	40	44	47	51	55	58	62
12	26	29	33	37	41	45	49	53	57	61	65	69
13	28	33	37	41	45	50	54	59	63	67	72	76
14	31	36	40	45	50	55	59	64	67	74	78	83
15	34	39	44	49	54	59	64	70	75	80	85	90
16	37	42	47	53	59	64	70	75	81	86	92	98
17	39	45	51	57	63	67	75	81	87	93	99	105
18	42	48	55	61	67	74	80	86	93	99	106	112
19	45	52	58	65	72	78	85	92	99	106	113	119
20	48	55	62	69	76	83	90	98	105	112	119	127

Table C.4. (continued)

c. One-tailed test when $\alpha = .05$; two-tailed test when $\alpha = .10$

N_1 \ N_2	9	10	11	12	13	14	15	16	17	18	19	20
1											0	0
2	1	1	1	2	2	2	3	3	3	4	4	4
3	3	4	5	5	6	7	7	8	9	9	10	11
4	6	7	8	9	10	11	12	14	15	16	17	18
5	9	11	12	13	15	16	18	19	20	22	23	25
6	12	14	16	17	19	21	23	25	26	28	30	32
7	15	17	19	21	24	26	28	30	33	35	37	39
8	18	20	23	26	28	31	33	36	39	41	44	47
9	21	24	27	30	33	36	39	42	45	48	51	54
10	24	27	31	34	37	41	44	48	51	55	58	62
11	27	31	34	38	42	46	50	54	57	61	65	69
12	30	34	38	42	47	51	55	60	64	68	72	77
13	33	37	42	47	51	56	61	65	70	75	80	84
14	36	41	46	51	56	61	66	71	77	82	87	92
15	39	44	50	55	61	66	72	77	83	88	94	100
16	42	48	54	60	65	71	77	83	89	95	101	107
17	45	51	57	64	70	77	83	89	96	102	109	115
18	48	55	61	68	75	82	88	95	102	109	116	123
19	51	58	65	72	80	87	94	101	109	116	123	130
20	54	62	69	77	84	92	100	107	115	123	130	138

Source: As adapted from D. Auble, "Extended Tables for the Mann-Whitney Statistic" *Bulletin of the Institute of Educational Research at Indiana University,* 1, 1953 by Sidney Siegel, *Nonparametric Statistics for the Behavioral Sciences,* 1956. Reprinted with permission of the authors, Indiana University, and McGraw-Hill Book Company.

How to Use Table C.5

If this table is used, the values of both n_1 and n_2 must be between 2 and 20. Table C.5 lists *maximum* r values in the Wald-Wolfowitz test for rejecting H_0 at the .05 level of significance. To find this value locate the n_2 value of interest among the values listed across the top of the table. Locate the n_1 value of interest among the values listed in the stub (far left) column of the table. Locate the intersection of the n_2 column and the n_1 row in the body of the table. Compare this table value with the calculated r value. If the calculated r value is *equal to or smaller than* the table value, *reject* H_0. If the calculated r is *greater than* the table value, *accept* H_0.

Example 1

H_1: Always nondirectional
α: .05
$n_1 = 8, n_2 = 11$
$r = 5$

Inference Decision

Reject H_0, since r of 5 is *equal to* table value of 5.

Statistical Tables

Table C.5. Maximum Values of r in Wald-Wolfowitz Test to Reject H_0 at $\alpha = .05$

n_1 \ n_2	2	3	4	5	6	7	8	9	10	11	12	13	14	15	16	17	18	19	20
2											2	2	2	2	2	2	2	2	2
3					2	2	2	2	2	2	2	2	2	3	3	3	3	3	3
4			2	2	2	2	3	3	3	3	3	3	3	3	4	4	4	4	4
5			2	2	3	3	3	3	3	4	4	4	4	4	4	4	5	5	5
6		2	2	3	3	3	3	4	4	4	4	5	5	5	5	5	5	6	6
7		2	2	3	3	3	4	4	5	5	5	5	5	6	6	6	6	6	6
8		2	3	3	3	4	4	5	5	5	6	6	6	6	6	7	7	7	7
9		2	3	3	4	4	5	5	5	6	6	6	7	7	7	7	8	8	8
10		2	3	3	4	5	5	5	6	6	7	7	7	7	8	8	8	8	9
11		2	3	4	4	5	5	6	6	7	7	7	8	8	9	9	9	9	9
12	2	2	3	4	4	5	6	6	7	7	7	8	8	8	9	9	9	10	10
13	2	2	3	4	5	5	6	6	7	7	8	8	9	9	9	10	10	10	10
14	2	2	3	4	5	5	6	7	7	8	8	9	9	9	10	10	10	11	11
15	2	3	3	4	5	6	6	7	7	8	8	9	9	10	10	11	11	11	12
16	2	3	4	4	5	6	6	7	8	9	9	9	10	10	11	11	11	12	12
17	2	3	4	4	5	6	7	7	8	9	9	10	10	11	11	11	12	12	13
18	2	3	4	5	5	6	7	8	8	9	9	10	10	11	11	12	12	13	13
19	2	3	4	5	6	6	7	8	8	9	10	10	11	11	12	12	13	13	13
20	2	3	4	5	6	6	7	8	9	9	10	10	11	12	12	13	13	13	14

Source: As adapted from Frieda S. Swed and C. Eisenhart, "Tables for Testing Randomness of Grouping in a Sequence of Alternatives," *Annals of Mathematical Statistics*, 14, 1943 by Sidney Siegel, *Nonparametric Statistics for the Behavioral Sciences*, 1956. Reprinted with permission of the authors, *Annals of Mathematical Statistics*, and McGraw-Hill Book Company.

Example 2

Inference Decision

H_1: Always nondirectional
α: .05
$n_1 = 17, n_2 = 13$
$r = 8$

Reject H_0, since r of 8 is *smaller than* table value of 10.

Example 3

Inference Decision

H_1: Always nondirectional
α: .05
$n_1 = 10, n_2 = 8$
$r = 7$

Accept H_0, since r of 7 is *greater than* table value of 5.

How to Use Table C.6

Locate degrees of freedom (df) at left and level of significance, according to whether a one- or two-tailed test is being
applied, at the top. The minimum t value required to reject
H_0 is listed at the intersection of that row and column.
For a one-tailed test predicting a negative t value (i.e., H_1:
$\overline{X}_1 < \overline{X}_2$) assign a negative sign to the t value obtained
from Table C.6. For a two-tailed test, two t values are re-
quired, one positive and one negative.

Example 1

df $= 18$

$H_1 : \overline{X}_1 > \overline{X}_2$

$\alpha = .05$

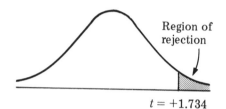

Region of
rejection

$t = +1.734$

Example 2

df $= 22$

$H_1 : \overline{X}_1 < \overline{X}_2$

$\alpha = .01$

Region of
rejection

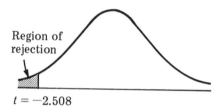

$t = -2.508$

Example 3

df $= 18$

$H_1 : \overline{X}_1 \neq \overline{X}_2$

$\alpha = .05$

Region of rejection

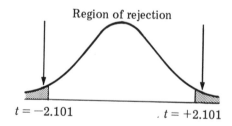

$t = -2.101$ $.\ t = +2.101$

Table C.6. Minimum Values of t to Reject H_0

df	Level of significance for one-tailed test					
	.10	.05	.025	.01	.005	.0005
	Level of significance for two-tailed test					
	.20	.10	.05	.02	.01	.001
1	3.078	6.314	12.706	31.821	63.657	636.619
2	1.886	2.920	4.303	6.965	9.925	31.598
3	1.638	2.353	3.182	4.541	5.841	12.941
4	1.533	2.132	2.776	3.747	4.604	8.610
5	1.476	2.015	2.571	3.365	4.032	6.859
6	1.440	1.943	2.447	3.143	3.707	5.959
7	1.415	1.895	2.365	2.998	3.499	5.405
8	1.397	1.860	2.306	2.896	3.355	5.041
9	1.383	1.833	2.262	2.821	3.250	4.781
10	1.372	1.812	2.228	2.764	3.169	4.587
11	1.363	1.796	2.201	2.718	3.106	4.437
12	1.356	1.782	2.179	2.681	3.055	4.318
13	1.350	1.771	2.160	2.650	3.012	4.221
14	1.345	1.761	2.145	2.624	2.977	4.140
15	1.341	1.753	2.131	2.602	2.947	4.073
16	1.337	1.746	2.120	2.583	2.921	4.015
17	1.333	1.740	2.110	2.567	2.898	3.965
18	1.330	1.734	2.101	2.552	2.878	3.922
19	1.328	1.729	2.093	2.539	2.861	3.883
20	1.325	1.725	2.086	2.528	2.845	3.850
21	1.323	1.721	2.080	2.518	2.831	3.819
22	1.321	1.717	2.074	2.508	2.819	3.792
23	1.319	1.714	2.069	2.500	2.807	3.767
24	1.318	1.711	2.064	2.492	2.797	3.745
25	1.316	1.708	2.060	2.485	2.787	3.725
26	1.315	1.706	2.056	2.479	2.779	3.707
27	1.314	1.703	2.052	2.473	2.771	3.690
28	1.313	1.701	2.048	2.467	2.763	3.674
29	1.311	1.699	2.045	2.462	2.756	3.659
30	1.310	1.697	2.042	2.457	2.750	3.646
40	1.303	1.684	2.021	2.423	2.704	3.551
60	1.296	1.671	2.000	2.390	2.660	3.460
120	1.289	1.658	1.980	2.358	2.617	3.373
∞	1.282	1.645	1.960	2.326	2.576	3.291

Source: Fisher and Yates, *Statistical Tables for Biological, Agricultural and Medical Research*, 1948. Reprinted with permission of the authors and Longman Group, Ltd., London.

How to Use Table C.7

Locate degrees of freedom (df) at left and level of significance, according to whether a one- or two-tailed test is being applied, at the top. The minimum Pearson's r value to reject H_0 is listed at the intersection of that row and column. For a one-tailed test predicting a negative r value (i.e., $H_1 : r < 0$), assign a negative sign to the r value obtained from Table C.7. For a two-tailed test, two r values are required, one positive and one negative.

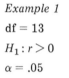

Example 1

df = 13

$H_1 : r > 0$

$\alpha = .05$

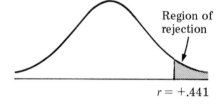

Region of rejection

$r = +.441$

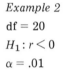

Example 2

df = 20

$H_1 : r < 0$

$\alpha = .01$

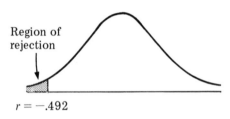

Region of rejection

$r = -.492$

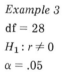

Example 3

df = 28

$H_1 : r \neq 0$

$\alpha = .05$

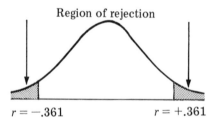

Region of rejection

$r = -.361$ $r = +.361$

When df > 48, r may be converted into a z score according to the formula $z = r\sqrt{N-1}$. Significance is then determined by reference to Table C.2.

Table C.7. Minimum Values of Pearson's r to Reject H_0.

	Level of significance for a directional (one-tailed) test				
	.05	.025	.01	.005	.0005
	Level of significance for a non-directional (two-tailed) test				
df = $N-2$	.10	.05	.02	.01	.001
1	.9877	.9969	.9995	.9999	1.0000
2	.9000	.9500	.9800	.9900	.9990
3	.8054	.8783	.9343	.9587	.9912
4	.7293	.8114	.8822	.9172	.9741
5	.6694	.7545	.8329	.8745	.9507
6	.6215	.7067	.7887	.8343	.9249
7	.5822	.6664	.7498	.7977	.8982
8	.5494	.6319	.7155	.7646	.8721
9	.5214	.6021	.6851	.7348	.8471
10	.4973	.5760	.6581	.7079	.8233
11	.4762	.5529	.6339	.6835	.8010
12	.4575	.5324	.6120	.6614	.7800
13	.4409	.5139	.5923	.6411	.7603
14	.4259	.4973	.5742	.6226	.7420
15	.4124	.4821	.5577	.6055	.7246
16	.4000	.4683	.5425	.5897	.7084
17	.3887	.4555	.5285	.5751	.6932
18	.3783	.4438	.5155	.5614	.6787
19	.3687	.4329	.5034	.5487	.6652
20	.3598	.4227	.4921	.5368	.6524
25	.3233	.3809	.4451	.4869	.5974
30	.2960	.3494	.4093	.4487	.5541
35	.2746	.3246	.3810	.4182	.5189
40	.2573	.3044	.3578	.3932	.4896
45	.2428	.2875	.3384	.3721	.4648
50	.2306	.2732	.3218	.3541	.4433
60	.2108	.2500	.2948	.3248	.4078
70	.1954	.2319	.2737	.3017	.3799
80	.1829	.2172	.2565	.2830	.3568
90	.1726	.2050	.2422	.2673	.3375
100	.1638	.1946	.2301	.2540	.3211

Source: Robert E. Gehring, *Basic Behavioral Statistics*, 1978. Reprinted with permission of the author and Houghton Mifflin Company.

Index

Index